T0227803

THE PSYCHOLOGY OF A
MUSICAL PRODIGY

Founded by C. K. Ogden

The International Library of Psychology

COGNITIVE PSYCHOLOGY
In 21 Volumes

THE PSYCHOLOGY OF A MUSICAL PRODIGY

G RÉVÉSZ

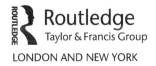

Routledge
Taylor & Francis Group

LONDON AND NEW YORK

First published in 1925 by
Routledge, Trench, Trubner & Co., Ltd.
2 Park Square, Milton Park, Abingdon, Oxfordshire OX14 4RN
711 Third Avenue, New York, NY 10017

First issued in paperback 2014

Routledge is an imprint of the Taylor and Francis Group, an informa business

© 1925 G Révész

British Library Cataloguing in Publication Data
A CIP catalogue record for this book
is available from the British Library

The Psychology of a Musical Prodigy
ISBN 0415-20970-6
Cognitive Psychology: 21 Volumes
ISBN 0415-21126-3
The International Library of Psychology: 204 Volumes
ISBN 0415-19132-7

ISBN 13: 978-1-138-87503-6 (pbk)
ISBN 13: 978-0-415-20970-0 (hbk)

CONTENTS

PREFACE

THIS work, the first of its kind, is an attempt to portray the development of a richly endowed artist, from his earliest youth up to a certain definite period of his existence, to analyse his artistic and intellectual capabilities, and to unite these into an integral whole.

There have been works without number dealing with the youth of artists, and the craze for the telling of anecdotes and the recording and inventing of peculiarities, has served to add to their profusion, until a more than sufficient record of the development of great men has been bequeathed to us. This record also includes many of their very early works. But, even if these traditions were authenticated in a more trustworthy manner than they usually are, they are disconnected and full of gaps, and cannot be compared with a careful observation of a single artistic personality, carried out with due regard to all the essential phenomena.

The same holds good of works dealing primarily with premature artistic development. Here, also, a continuous record of artistic creation, as revealed to us by the close observation of creative activity, affords us an insight into artistic development, which is important not only for the elucidation of the problem of the particular individuality concerned, but also for establishing general principles of artistic creation.

I am of the opinion that the systematic investigation of the development of a highly-gifted child will ensure us a better understanding of the phenomena with which we are confronted in the early artistic growth of many artists. These phenomena, mysterious so long as they are isolated, become indispensable as soon as they are linked up and incorporated into a whole. Whether such an aim will be attained, depends, on the one hand, on the method and scope of investigation, and, on the other, on the attitude of the investigator, who must be able, to a certain extent, to relinquish preconceived views and prejudices. To every investigator the thought must always be present, that the character which he is observing is that of another individual, and differs therein from his own, and that his comprehension of it, though extensive, must always remain limited ; he must also always remember that his own experiences are largely incomplete, and that the material at his command is fragmentary, and only where these fragments are brought into proper combination will the inner nature of the artist be revealed to us with clearness and precision.

In this work I have endeavoured to put before the public the result of my researches on the mentality of an unusually gifted child. If I have been successful in selecting, from among a number of observations, those which are most characteristic and which serve to complete the picture of little Erwin, I may perhaps have succeeded in throwing some light on the great mystery of evolution. In connection with this, I will deal with some problems relative to my particular subject, such as, for instance, the appearance of musical talent at an early age, the theory of musical genius, the different aspects of musical talent and their investigation, etc. The book has been written and the subject treated in such a manner as to provide a psychological interest for people who have no close connection with music. I do not consider that these observations on the progress of development of one child in particular point to anything psychologically unique in my model, but I see in him, apart from certain individual traits, a typical example of one kind of musical artistic development. Therefore I am of the opinion that the present investigation may prove historically useful, and that, by assuming that a similar course of development has taken place in the early lives of some of the famous musicians, certain hiatuses may be covered, and many doubtful points explained.

Finally, I have printed a small selection of Erwin's compositions that musical readers may follow his progress in creative activity by observing his creations themselves. Thus, perhaps, words and music may be successful in achieving what words without music, and music without words, would fail to convey.

G. RÉVÉSZ

AMSTERDAM, *November* 1924.

THE PSYCHOLOGY OF A MUSICAL PRODIGY

1. Introductory

MODERN psychology, for some time past, has over-stepped its initial programme, and has outgrown the scope of the intentions and hopes originally formulated by Fechner. The methods of investigation have become more varied, new fields have been opened, and prob-lems have been attacked which were formerly regarded as inaccessible to exact research. The processes of psychic activity are being investigated with more and more precision, and attempts are also being made to analyse complicated psychic structures. We are no longer content to establish general laws; personality itself, individually and in its development, is already being made the subject of inquiry. As innate ten-dencies are of fundamental importance in the evolution of personality, it is of particular advantage to undertake researches of this kind in the case of persons who show themselves already in their early youth to be endowed in an extraordinary measure with spiritual or artistic capabilities.

I found myself in touch with a temperament which appeared to me to be of the highest interest from the

A

point of view of musical art, in the person of a child whose psychic life I tried to study more closely.

On first meeting this remarkable child I had a strong impression that I was in the presence of a most interesting case, and I therefore profited by the occasion, one which rarely presents itself to a psychologist, to carry out a systematic observation of an "infant prodigy".

Such research is apt to give us, on the one hand, information as to certain phenomena, such as the relations and operations of the laws characteristic of artistic creation ; on the other hand it may lead us to certain conclusions with regard to the course of evolution usually taken by artistic talent. The insight which we obtain during research of this kind may often be of service in solving the universal problems that arise in connection with artistic production. Such an inquiry may also enlighten us as to what rôle is played by innate and inherited tendencies, a subject the deepest roots of which have not yet been tapped, and may help us to determine the mental and artistic capabilities of human endeavour.

I have examined this extraordinarily gifted child, with the aid of the methods at my disposal, endeavouring to discover the extent of his mental capacity and endowment, and, in connection with this, to establish what influences determined the development of his musical talent.

If, as time goes on, other similar cases are subjected to minute investigation, it will be possible to compare the different personalities with each other, having regard to their capacities, their development, etc., and, as a result, it will be possible to realize more clearly the importance of many events and phases in the complicated course of development of the artist.

In the present work I have, I believe, been the first to attempt the investigation of the mental growth of a particularly gifted person during the most interesting and enlightening period of his evolution, and to follow the unfolding of a striking gift from the very beginnings until the end of its first period of development. In spite of the difficulties that naturally arise in a field in which, up to now, no principles for systematic work have been established, I hope that the method I have adopted for the solution of the various problems and in the investigation of mental and artistic attributes, added to the diverse points of view from which I have regarded this temperament, may help others who may undertake similar research.

The subject of my investigations, Erwin Nyiregyházi, is already a famous pianist, and was, at that time, a child of great talent as a composer, and endowed with a remarkable capacity for musical interpretation.

His personality as a child bore a marked resemblance to that of the infant Mozart. His creative gift, awakened at an early age, his general premature development, the keenness and ease of his creative ability, the rapidity of his artistic evolution, his remarkable talent for instrumental technique, his great love of art, as well as his intelligence, which is above the normal level, his wit, his joy in life, his tenderness, his devotion to his parents, and, finally, his attachment to his teachers, are all of them features which are inseparable from the picture of the child Mozart.

As early as in the spring of 1910 I was engaged in the examination of Erwin, and would have liked to publish the results of my investigation in that year. Except, however, for a short report, which I submitted to the Congress for Experimental Psychology at Innsbruck in April 1910, I did not publish anything on the results of my researches. I decided to keep the child under systematic observation during a longer period of his mental and artistic development, in view of the fact that, during the three ensuing years, his musical talents developed in an unusual manner, especially his gift for composition, which expanded in such a measure that my hope of seeing Erwin become a great artist was justified. It is owing to this delay in the publication of my observations that I am now enabled to add to my earlier notes a series of more recent investigations concerning the development of the child in the three ensuing years.

I will now proceed to give a short account of Erwin's life, since the influence of his home and that of the circumstances under which he lived, seem to me to play a part of some importance in his development.

2. Life of Erwin Nyiregyházi

ERWIN NYIREGYHÁZI was born at Budapest, on the 19th of January 1903. His parents belonged to the educated middle classes, his father, as well as his grandfather on the father's side, being tenor singers in the chorus of the Royal Opera of Budapest. The family, therefore, had been connected with music for the last two generations. Indeed his father, although unable to devote himself to a more thorough study of the art, being obliged to work for his living, and having risen gradually from very poor circumstances, had, nevertheless, a deeper understanding of musical matters than is usually found in chorus singers. Erwin's mother also possessed considerable musical talent and appears to have been a better musician than the father; he, on the other hand, seems to have had a more intimate inner relation to music than his wife. It may therefore be said that Erwin owes his musical talent, in so far as it may be considered an inheritance, to his parents.[1] If it were feasible in this case to employ the genealogical method, and trace the musical record of Erwin's forbears, it might be possible to ascertain to which line of ancestors the transmission of inherited musical

---

[1] It is remarkable that musical talent is to be found also in the younger son of the Nyiregyházi family, who, at the time of writing this book, was five years old. The little boy was remarkable for a strong feeling of rhythm, and a very good musical memory.

ability is particularly to be ascribed. But this, to our regret, is impossible, and we must confine our researches to their still living descendants, as the only data concerning the previous history of the family, which I have been able to obtain by questioning some of its members, are regrettably vague and, in fact, extend only to the immediately preceding generation.

In spite of careful research all that I could discover concerning the Nyiregyházi family was that a near relative of the father's mother used to teach the piano in a small provincial town, and that, among the ancestors of the father, there were a number of distinguished ecclesiastics, whose mental qualities certainly show themselves in Erwin.

If it were not established that the grandfather on the father's side was a musician ; if, therefore, musical talent, even in a slight degree, did not manifest itself in the father and grandfather ; if, further, the biographies of famous musicians did not tend to show that, in the great majority of cases, the inheritance of artistic talent is derived from the father, one might feel inclined, owing to the greater talent of the mother, to ascribe the musical ability of Erwin to the maternal influence. The case would not be an isolated one, for many instances are known, illustrating the transmission of musical talent through the maternal side, as in the case of Mendelssohn, Grieg, Gounod, Rubinstein, and others.[1]

The chief interest of the parents was at that time centred in the boy, in whom they saw a future maestro. It is greatly to be regretted that the father died early,

[1] Compare this with Th. Ribot, *L'hérédité psychologique*, Paris, 1893.

and that thus the child lost his chief support in life. We owe it to his memory to record the fact that he wished to secure for the boy a quiet and undisturbed period of training. He was far from desiring, as often happens in the case of the fathers of "child prodigies", to exploit his son's talent as a means of subsistence for the whole family, but, on the contrary, did everything in his power to assist him to become not only a fine, but a thoroughly well-trained artist.

Concerning the progress of the development of Erwin's talent I can furnish the following information :

Erwin was not one year old when he tried to imitate singing. Of this his father is witness. In the second year of his life he is said to have already been able to reproduce correctly melodies sung to him at a time when his capacity for verbal expression was, of course, still very poor and defective.[1] Indeed, as the parents report, the development of speech was, in the case of Erwin, actually retarded, so that a decided progress in this respect was only noticeable in the third year of his age. The actual form of this retarded development of speech I was not able definitely to ascertain. I have received data on this subject, but they were too unreliable to enable me to form from them a clear impression of the development of Erwin's speech. We must, therefore, be satisfied with the important fact that, even before the period of proper development of speech, the vocal reproduction of heard melodies was accomplished by Erwin without difficulty.

---

[1] Of Handel also it is said that he sang at an age when he was still unable to speak.

When he had completed his third year his father had already discovered that the child had a sense of absolute pitch, and he could correctly locate on the piano notes that were sung to him.[1] According to the evidence both of his parents and their friends, Erwin was able to reproduce any melody sung to him with exactness on the mouth-organ.

At the beginning of his fourth year he began to play on the piano everything that he had heard. During this time his talent for composition began to show itself in improvising and playing stray fragments he had invented. When he was three and a half years old he already composed little melodies, with accompaniment. As I have been informed, he played his own compositions before the celebrated 'cellist, David Popper, and before Julius Erkel, both professors of music at the Musical Academy, in 1907, that is to say, in his fifth year. Up to this time Erwin had not received any instruction in music, and it was only in his fifth year that he was given lessons in piano-playing and reading of music. At first, indeed, the teaching was irregular, and was received with little seriousness by the pupil, and, only in his sixth year, when he was entered as a student at the Academy of Music, did his regular tuition in music begin. From his sixth until his twelfth year, at which time I was obliged to give up my observations, owing to his departure from his native land, his life took a normal course. Music was

---

[1] It would, of course, have been possible to observe his gift of perfect pitch earlier, as it was inborn. It may be noticed that neither his parents nor his grandfather possessed this faculty.

the centre of his interest during this time, to which there was gradually added an intense wish on his part to acquire information on all possible subjects. School did not satisfy his thirst for knowledge : he employed all the means at his disposal in order to follow his many-sided interests. The lasting effect of these activities manifested themselves later in intellectual prowess.

From a musical standpoint this was a felicitous period for Erwin. In creative and, more especially, in interpretative art, he developed beyond all expectation. At this time he had not begun to play at public concerts, but, in his performances before musicians, his success was frequent, both in his own country and abroad. He went once, by invitation, to London, where he played before the Royal family, and, in the house of Mr Asquith, then Prime Minister, before a select public.

His creative activity, in the proper sense of the word, had already begun in his sixth year. At this time his first written pieces were composed, such as a barcarole, a berceuse, a dance of elves, a wedding march (the only work published before his twelfth year), a funeral march, for 'cello, and, finally, a serenata, certain of which I publish in the Appendix. Though his remarkable creative genius only declared itself later, these pieces already clearly show a most distinct talent for composition. But a considerable length of time passed before he began to study harmony, this theoretical musical instruction only lasting a short time, being cut short, owing to external causes, after fifteen lessons, and not until a year later did he take it up again. From this time onward, Erwin pursued his studies regularly with only a few interruptions, varying in length.[1] I shall give a more detailed account of this and of the various phases of his musical development in another chapter.

As the years passed, the external conditions of his life assumed a more and more favourable aspect. The family were comfortably off and their means, combined with the active interest taken by their friends in the boy's career, made it unnecessary for them to place any restrictions on his musical training.

Erwin was, therefore, in a position to devote himself unhampered to his art; he had been saved both from poverty and from great wealth, the two disastrous extremes on the economic scale. As regards the artistic *milieu* of Erwin it may be mentioned that he missed the special privilege of maturing under the stimulating influence of a musical home and artistic surroundings. It cannot, indeed, be said that the absence of such surroundings exercises any adverse influence on the development of his talent, which unfolded most rapidly and flowered at a very early age; still, it may be safely assumed that the stimulus which an artistic *milieu*, and specially that of a musical family, usually gives, would certainly have been beneficial to his development as an artist.

[1] At Budapest his tuition in piano-playing was placed in the hands of the pianist Székely; composition was taught to him first by Siklós, later on by the well-known composer, L. Weiner, both of them teachers at the Royal Academy of Music. When the boy moved to Berlin in 1914 his musical education was pursued by the renowned pianist, E. v. Dohnányi, and by the conductors, M. Fiedler and S. Ochs, with great devotion. After a series of concerts, at which he performed in Europe, he went, a few years ago, to America, where he is now playing.

3. On the Early Appearance of Musical Talent in General

It is evident that, in this case, we have to deal with a boy endowed with musical interpretative and creative gifts. That the talent for composition should show itself in so marked a manner so early in life—in fact, almost in infancy, and *before the power of interpretation*, makes our case appear all the more remarkable, since it is well-known that such juvenile composers are rarely met with. Indeed, that creative talent should appear at all at such an early age, is quite exceptional.

As a rule, in the case of so-called "infant prodigies," interpretative artistic talent appears occasionally as early as before the child's eighth year; the gift for composition, on the other hand, in the great majority of cases, is observed only when childhood is drawing to a close. The fact that the power of interpretation shows itself earlier than the creative power [1] explains why children with creative as well as interpretative ability, usually appear before the public as executants much earlier than as composers. They are, therefore, in the

---

[1] Generally speaking, technically and artistically - technical capabilities appear at an earlier age than creative capabilities. These are the forms of talent which have the closest relation to emotional and instinctive life, and are less closely related to intellectual development in its proper sense. See for particulars, my paper: *Das frühzeitige Auftreten der Begabung und ihre Erkennung* (Premature Appearance of Talent), Leipzig, 1921.

first period of their musical activity, admired as virtuosos, whereas the modest utterances of their creative gift are hardly ever considered as deserving of notice.

Thus, in the case of J. S. Bach, we know that he had mastered the technique of both the violin and the organ, while his creative talent only awakened at a comparatively late period. During his life at Ohrdruff (from his tenth to his fourteenth year) he is not known, with certainty, to have composed at all, though it might be possible to assign the still very primitive fugue in E minor (unpublished) to this period.[1] It was not until his eighteenth year that he produced some works for the organ, which have become known. It is true that the inventive faculty of Bach must have been fostered at an early age by the playing of thorough-bass and the extemporizing of preludes, but whether this resulted in any original compositions, it is not possible to determine.

In the case of Handel the creative instinct was not apparent in early youth or at the beginning of his musical career, but only manifested itself after a comparatively long period, during which he received continuous instruction in music. He was already well-known as an organ-player at the age of eight, whereas his first compositions of any importance date from his eleventh year. There are, however, students of musical history who assign the six sonatas, or trios, for two oboes and bass, which are usually attributed to his eleventh year, to a later period.[2]

[1] R. Batka, *J. S. Bach*, Leipzig, 1892, p. 34.
[2] V. Schölcher, *The Life of Handel*, London, 1857.

The first compositions of Beethoven date from his twelfth and thirteenth years. So much, at least, is certain, that he himself declared the *Variations in minor keys*, and the three *Sonatas* composed in 1783 (he was born 1770) to have been his earliest works.[1] It is also an established fact that his great gift as a composer only developed in the year 1792, after his removal to Vienna. The time of apprenticeship served by him in Bonn gave no opportunity for the recognition of his genius, and, at that time, he was merely considered an excellent improvisatore, and a very good player of thorough-bass. Of the compositions produced in Bonn, a great number, according to the opinion of his biographers, were later printed with a higher *opus* number than the first of the works composed in Vienna; but they show a marked deficiency in value compared with the early Viennese publications. In fact, Beethoven, during the Bonn period, had not yet come before the public as a composer to any important extent; he was still in the student stage, intent on preparing himself for future achievements.[2]

As regards Mendelssohn, it is true that he began composing at an early age, but not before he was ten. Lampadius, his excellent biographer, gives an account of a fugue which is said to have been composed by him at the age of eleven. In the case of Mendelssohn, it is not so much the exceptionally early appearance of his creative talent as the great speed of its development

---

[1] A. B. Marx, *L. v. Beethoven*, vol. 2, Appendix II, p. 512.
[2] H. Riemann, *Geschichte der Musik seit Beethoven*, Berlin, 1901, p. 52.

and his enormous capacity for production, which call for admiration. He was not twelve years old when he composed his first *opera*, and in his thirteenth year he had already produced a large number of musical works very varied in character.[1]

In the case of Brahms also, the talent for instrumental technique showed itself at a much earlier date than that for composition. All the same, we know that his first attempts at creative work took place early, between his tenth and twelfth year, as his piano teacher complained, during this period, of the boy's unbridled habit of composing. So much is certain that, at the age of thirteen, he had written a song for a Male Vocal Society and that, in 1849, when he was sixteen, he performed a fantasy of his own on a popular waltz at his second concert. His first real work, however, the *Sonata in F sharp minor*, was not written till 1852.[2]

Cherubini, Spohr, Löwe, Berlioz, Bruckner, Tchaikovsky[3] gave evidence of creative talent at an early age, but not in extreme youth.

Haydn is one of the few great musicians who, besides showing marked capacity as a pianist, showed signs of marked creative faculty at a very early age, beginning, in fact, to compose when he was six years old.

This is also apparent in the musical development of Mozart, of whom it is said that he had already composed piano pieces before the age of six. It is a matter for regret that these pieces have not come down to us.

[1] W. A. Lampadius, *Felix Mendelssohn-Bartholdy*, Leipzig, 1886.
[2] W. A. Thomas-San-Galli, *Johannes Brahms*, Munich, 1912.
[3] O. Feis, *Studien über die Geneologie und Psychologie der Musiker*, Wiesbaden, 1910, p. 21.

It is probable that they were never committed to paper. We know of a series of minuets, dating from his sixth year, which are distinguished by the formal purity of their style, simplicity and clearness of melody, and which point to the presence of a great creative talent. The *Minuet in F major*, dated 11th May, and the minuet set to the same bass, dated July 1762, are particularly successful. In the year 1764, when he was eight years old, he had already produced six sonatas for the piano and the violin, and three symphonies for small orchestra.[1]

Schubert is said to have written quite a number of songs and pieces for the piano before his tenth year. At any rate it is certain that the attention of Salieri, an influential orchestra conductor in Vienna, had been drawn to the genius of the young Schubert as early as 1811, by his song "The Complaint of Hagar." His rapid advance as a composer and his enormous productivity is as wonderful as that of Mendelssohn. In 1815 he composed a number of works for the stage, masses, sonatas for the piano, and about one hundred and seventy songs.[2]

The talent for composition also showed itself at an early age in the case of Chopin. He is said to have produced pieces for the piano as early as at the age of eight. His first publications, however, did not appear until later. His *Opus* 1, the *Rondo in C minor* dates from the year 1827, when he was seventeen years of

[1] O. Jahn, *W. A. Mozart*, Fourth ed. 1905-1907 ; L. v. Köchel, *Chronologisch-thematisches Verzeichnis sämtlicher Tonwerke W. A. Mozarts*, Leipzig, 1862.
[2] H. Riemann, loc. cit. p. 122 ff.

age. At this time, however, he had already given public performances of quite a number of admirable compositions, which were not published till a later date. In his twentieth year, during his stay in Vienna and Paris, Chopin was already a perfectly matured composer, whose individual character was definitely formed.[1]

In the case of Meyerbeer, the creative aspect of his talent found expression at a very early age. Even before his tenth year he is said to have composed a considerable number of vocal and piano pieces. His gift for instrumental technique appeared at a much earlier date.

As regards Camille Saint-Saëns it is reported that his creative activity began at the age of five; and of Richard Strauss that he commenced composing at the age of six; his work at this period being, however, unknown.

Thus the biography of the great composers teaches us that, as opposed to interpretative artistic talent, the gift for composition only shows itself during early childhood in the very rarest cases. It must always be looked upon as an exception, when a child surprises us with creative ability in extreme youth, at a time when his creative powers ought still to be subservient to his bodily and mental evolution, and should be sufficiently occupied by this in itself. It is for this reason that the case which I describe here is of such particular interest, because in it we see, in the creative efforts of a little child, a sound and genuine capacity to give form to thoughts and emotions. In spite of insufficient instruc-

[1] H. Leichentritt, *Friedr. Chopin*, Berlin, 1905.

tion and a complete lack of knowledge concerning the theory of composition, we see musical thoughts already taking form, and becoming musical units of high order, as I shall have occasion to show in greater detail when discussing the child's compositions.

I do not, in this work, propose to inquire more deeply into the significance of the fact that productive talent should appear at so early an age, for this would necessitate a preliminary inquiry into a number of problems. It would, indeed, be necessary to make a thorough analysis of artistic, and more especially of musical tendencies, in addition to a more thorough inquiry into the special nature of music.

That musical talent, and particularly the creative side of the gift for music, may appear unmistakably in early childhood, and that, in some cases, it even leads to really artistic productions—a phenomenon which has not, until now, been observed in other branches of art[1]—is no doubt due, to a certain extent, to the nature of music itself, and will admit of this explanation. It also points towards the fact that the gift for music does not seem to be so closely dependent on the mental level of the inspired person, as is the case in other arts, assuming that level to be a normal one.[2] It also would

---

[1] Raphael, whose artistic genius appeared at an unusually early age, only painted his first important pictures at the ages of fifteen and sixteen. These, however, were still so strongly under the influence of his master Perugino, that, according to Vasari's testimony, it was impossible to distinguish them from Perugino's own works.

[2] By this I do not mean that the intellectual development of a musician may have no influence on his musical creations, or that the solution of some artistic problems may not presuppose a highly-developed intellect of a particular kind.

B

appear that music depends less than other arts on general mental development. A young child, still at the beginning of his mental evolution, may already be possessed of a rich creative genius. It would seem that the evolution of musical talent is dependent rather on certain biological conditions in the individual, a view towards which we are inclined by the fact that, in almost every case, the talent for music manifests itself very strongly between the ages of thirteen and fifteen, at a time at which the main period of bodily development has just closed, and the mental faculties proper are usually still very far from being fully developed.

That creative musical talent should appear at such an early age prompts us, further, to surmise that musical invention stands in less close relation to experience and practice than creative activity in the other arts, and above all in science. This may, in great part, be explained by the fact that music does not take its subject-matter from nature; it does not draw upon what the artist receives during his life, is not fed from the outer world, and is hardly ever stimulated by it, but is nourished from *within*. External experience lends very little to it, for neither its form nor its substance stands in any close relation to the sensual world or the objects of sensual experience; no other art draws its rules, its principles and its material so entirely from itself, and none of them is, in its development, so independent of other arts, or to a certain extent so independent of technique (popular songs) as music. And it is for this reason that music is the most personal of all the arts; that is why, during the enjoyment of music, one keeps oneself apart from all the impressions of the material world ; one feels as if one were encompassed by an impervious veil ; one is absent-minded, deeply absorbed in the interior of the soul. But it would be incorrect to assume that music is so bound up with our feelings and emotions as to be properly regarded as the adequate expression of these—a view that has already been refuted by Hegel and Schopenhauer, and which has been embodied in the theories of music expressed by various students of æsthetics.[1] The emotions excited by music are *specifically musical* emotions, and, even if they are not of a purely musical character, the musical element in them is the element sustaining the whole. The differences that exist between these and other types of emotion will be made the subject of a separate inquiry in another work.[2] It is safe to assume that the emotions which precede musical creation and which are active in composition, are as a rule specifically musical in character. It will, therefore, be correct to assume that musical invention draws its material from an independent source, belonging exclusively to music. This independence explains why creative musical talent is not in close connection with the other mental qualities. This may also be observed in the case of a genius for mathematics, who feeds upon an entirely independent

[1] Compare E. Hanslick, *Vom Musikalisch - Schönen*, Leipzig, 1910, eleventh ed., p. 20 ff. ; P. Moos, *Die Philosophie der Musik*, Stuttgart, 1922.

[2] A very remarkable analysis of æsthetic enjoyment is to be found in M. Geiger's " Beiträge zur Phänomenologie des ästhetischen Genusses," *Jahrbuch für Philosophie und phänomenologische Forschung*, Vol. I, Halle, 1913, where, among other questions, the various psychic attitudes during musical enjoyment are treated with clear analytical insight.

and peculiar source, and herein lies the reason why, in this field, so important a part is played by hereditary transmission, why the capacity for and interest in this form of mental activity shows itself at such an early age, why a gift of this kind is so well-defined, why the division between mathematically-productive and mathematically - reproductive talent (creative and receptive capacity) is so marked, and why the development of this form of genius is so rapid.[1]

[1] The musical problems on which I have only touched cursorily in this chapter will be made the subject of a detailed inquiry in a book on subjects connected with the psychology of music, which will be published shortly in this Library. In that book I shall attempt to investigate the whole range of the problem of musical talent in relation to the general psychology of music.

4. On the General Aspect of Musical Talent

I PROPOSE now to record the development of Erwin's musical abilities and attributes during the period between the seventh and twelfth years of his life, and the gradual evolution of his talent for composition, up to and including his twelfth year, in order to give the reader as vivid a picture as possible of the child's genius.

Although, in this research, I am always primarily concerned with Erwin's talent, I should like, by a systematic investigation of the child's musical development, also to obtain data on the general laws which govern the evolution of musical genius. It will, however, be possible to penetrate more deeply into these laws when systematic investigation has been carried out on a number of unusually talented children.

Apart from his musical attributes, I shall pay special attention to the other mental qualities of Erwin, for it is impossible, in this particular instance, to give an adequate description of the child's personality, even of his musical characteristics alone, without taking into account his general mental qualities, his intelligence and his emotional and volitional life. And as, at the time, I was interested in his mental level as well as in his future development, I was of the opinion that I could obtain a broader basis for the prognostication of his future artistic development by a thorough knowledge of his general capacities.

The psychological examination of a musician has this advantage, compared to the study of other artists, that, in the case of the former, most of the musical artistic faculties and qualities, the thorough knowledge of which is essential in judging a musician's talent, may, up to a certain point, be reviewed singly, and the development of each of them may thus be made the subject of separate observation.

I propose to begin this investigation by examining "musicality" in general. It is, no doubt, difficult to define exactly what I would imply by this term. I can only give a general idea of my meaning by indicating the ways in which this quality expresses itself.

A close analysis of musicality, is, accordingly, a rather formidable task, for, on the one hand, it is difficult to give a precise definition of musicality and, on the other, the use made of this word is not a uniform one, as some people employ it in a narrower, others in a broader sense. Therefore, in order to make myself perfectly clear, it is necessary first to define the expression "musicality", which will occur so often in the course of my research, with as much precision as possible.[1] Musicality, primarily, denotes the ability to enjoy music æsthetically. Further, every degree of profound understanding of musical form and the structure of musical composition is based on musicality.

[1] Compare my paper, " Prüfung der Musikalität " (A Study of Musicality), *Zeitschrift für Psychologie*, 1920, vol. 85, pp. 163-207.

A musical person has a fine and developed instinct for the style and the rigid order of a musical sequence of ideas. Another necessary characteristic of a musical person is his capacity for becoming absorbed in the emotions expressed by music and his ability to enter into so intimate a relation with it, that the whole organization of his soul is affected. The possession of all these qualities results in a capacity for enjoyment which makes music part of the listener's very life, and gives him the power to judge and appreciate musical works of art according to their true value.

A musical person understands the marvel of artistic creation : he lives in it so thoroughly that he feels like a creator himself. A musical person experiences this act of creation, when engaged, purely æsthetically, in assimilating a work of musical art into his consciousness, just as strongly as when interpreting other people's compositions. He fills the creations of others, when listening to them or interpreting them, with the musical emotions experienced in his own soul; he understands them in his own personal way; and it is only through this vital activity of his own that he reaches the essence of a work of art.

Musicality is a fundamental entity like the " art sense " in the field of painting and sculpture. It cannot be evoked by education, it can only be developed; it is an innate and basic quality of the psychic organization of the person who possesses it, and it is a characteristic trait of his individuality. It finds expression, not only at times of æsthetic enjoyment, but also in the course of many other activities of life, which do not stand in any, or at least in no immediate, relation to music (as, for instance, in a man's relations with nature and poetry, and also in those which he creates between his musical experiences and emotional impressions of a different kind). All this serves to show that musicality is an essential factor, not only in the musical, but in the whole personality of man.

Musicality, as is seen in the foregoing short exposition, does not supply us with an instrument by which to estimate musical abilities, although it is always possible to form an unhesitating judgment as to whether a man is musical or not.

Other aspects of musical ability are more amenable to investigation; for instance, that which interests me particularly, the talent for *composition*. In order to analyse this, and to utilize it for drawing a complete picture of musical ability, it is necessary to collect compositions from various periods of development, and compare them with each other, and with the juvenile works of other composers. Thus may be ascertained the manner in which productive talent has developed in the course of years: whether the evolution was a continuous or an uncontinuous one; whether it ran parallel to the development of other mental faculties or not, or whether perhaps the various activities succeeded each other in their dominant rôle from time to time. The study of juvenile works also provides us with the necessary data in determining what influences have been of importance in the development of the corresponding mental faculties and, through them, may be traced the influence of the acquisition of certain kinds of knowledge, such as theoretical harmony and counterpoint, or the inspiration of composers with whom the child has come into intimate contact during his apprenticeship. The comparative study of juvenile works makes it possible to prognosticate the subsequent growth of the young artist by comparing his development with that of those great masters of music, who have been remarkable for premature creative talent.

In judging the musical talent of a child, his power of interpretation must also be taken into account. Careful distinction must, however, be made between mere precision and delicacy of technique, ease in overcoming difficulties, or, in short, cleverness and dexterity, on the one hand, and genuinely musical, inspired, and creative interpretation, on the other.

Genuine interpretation is, indeed, always a kind of creative faculty. The fact that reproductive talent is also, in its own way, creative, is shown most clearly when many kinds of original works, differing largely in character, are being interpreted. Reproductive ability, in the field of music as well as in that of the drama, may indeed rise to the highest summit of independent artistic achievement, and the interpretative work of a musical executant may well be compared to that of a great actor.

If, in the interpretation of musical creations, the aim to be attained were that of mere reproduction, such as the copying of a picture or a statue, it would be possible to point to one of many reproductions, as that which should be considered the most exact and faithful. But nothing of this kind is possible. Each of the great masters of the concert platform, as well as of the stage, interprets the same work in a different manner—they may even contradict each other up to a certain point, but each interpretation is perfect of its kind, and each gives expression to the greatness and beauty of the work. The great interpreters of musical and histrionic art are real magicians, who, from dumb forms and words, bring to light treasures which do not reveal themselves easily; they are the seers who look upon deep secrets, handed down to them by some inspired spirit, and bring them nearer to our understanding. Thus, it is not possible to say of any artist, however great, that he is better able to interpret the depth of a musical or poetic work, or that he does so in a manner more closely allied to the spirit of the author, than any other of the great artists who have endeavoured to solve the same problem. For every great artist interprets the work according to his own personality. The manner in which he understands the work, and the kind of interpretation he considers most suitable to it, spring from a necessity rooted in his own nature. In reproducing something, the artist shows himself, he gives expression to his own inner life. This particular kind of interpretation is embodied in his own person, and is his own original creation.

It is, therefore, of great importance in our judgment of an artist to determine whether his interpretation is based on mere external imitation or on his own understanding of the work; whether the artist is giving expression to the voice of another person or to his own.

There are cases, however, in which the study of

creative and interpretative forms of art is *insufficient* in formulating a judgment on the question of musical talent.   This is the case with musically gifted children, if they are still at the beginning of their artistic evolution, when their talent as composers and interpretative artists has not yet had a chance to unfold itself. In such cases a different method of gauging talent must be adopted, for it is necessary to be able to form a judgment on the capacity of such artists in the stage when it is still a mere *natural endowment*.   This end may best be attained if, instead of considering their various individual achievements, attention is concentrated on the amount of progress achieved, and further, if a study is also made of their elementary musical and acoustic abilities, observing these, also, as far as is possible, with regard to their development.   Finally, it is advisable to take impeding circumstances and the influence of hereditary transmission into account, since these are important if one would express a view on the magnitude of a musician's talent.

In any case, when investigating musical talent in its entirety, we must not omit general intelligence, which forms the foundation upon which all other gifts rest, and especially the acoustic faculties (the power of appreciating intervals, perfect pitch, musical memory).

Finally, sight must not be lost of the importance of education, of surroundings, of the intelligence of the parents, and, in general, of the intellectual level of those persons who have stood in immediate relationship to the child, and have had an influence on his intellectual development.

By investigating these subjects, we should be in a position, on the one hand, to obtain a more exact impression of the abilities of certain musical "infant prodigies" than is generally to be found in contemporaneous reports, and, on the other, to arrive at more detailed and more authentic information as to the fundamental characteristics of the "infant prodigy" in general. For our knowledge of the childhood of those artists who have been considered prodigies is very limited and not always to be relied upon. The greater part of such information usually consists of anecdotes or tradition by word of mouth, which generally has its source in juvenile memories, or in the reports of teachers and members of the artist's family. But these reports cannot always be trusted, even though they come from contemporary witnesses, the less so if they deal with individual occurrences, for, in this case, they are often obviously biased by affection. In most cases, indeed, they have not been written or told from a scientific standpoint, but are merely private, intimate communications, which, though they are founded on truth, do not on the whole strictly adhere to it. More detailed descriptions, such as, for instance, Richet's and Stumpf's treatises on the young violinist, Pepito Ariola, are, so far as I know, hardly to be found anywhere else.[1] Thus, very often during the study of Erwin, I was able to prove how little reports from people who are not trained psychologically are to be trusted. I had to

---

[1] Ch. Richet, "Note sur un cas remarquable de précocité musicale," *IV Congrès International de Psychologie*, Paris, 1900. *Compte-rendu des sciences*, Paris, 1901, pp. 93-99 ; Stumpf, "Akustische Versuche mit Pepito Ariola," *Zeitschrift f. angewandte Psychologie*, Vol. II, p. 1 ff.

check every piece of information before utilizing it.   It is characteristic of Erwin that, among all the data I received from various sources, those obtained from Erwin himself were those which corresponded most nearly to the truth.

The present inquiry is the first, and up to now has remained the only one, which shows the development of an "infant prodigy" in all its essential aspects, and attempts to build up, from individual data, the spiritual and artistic character of the child.

5. Diagnosis of Erwin's Mental Capacity by the aid of Tests

In order to obtain a general view of the child's mental capacity, I have endeavoured, as I have said before, thoroughly to ascertain the scope and degree of his general mental faculties, my chief task being to investigate his intelligence.

If we wish to estimate the degree of a child's intelligence we may adopt the method of addressing certain definite questions to him. In this way, we may assign to each child examined a more advanced, or a more backward, place in the scale of intelligence, according to how he answers these questions. It is well known that a standard representing what may be called the normal degree of development of the infantile mind has been established by formulating a certain series of mental tests corresponding to the average intellectual level of a certain age. If a child is able to give correct answers to questions which correspond to a more advanced age, it may be considered to be above normal, whereas if it is unable to answer the questions corresponding to its own age it must be classed as intellectually below the normal level.

Thus, each child may be said to be of a certain age as regards its intellectual development, this age being that which corresponds, in the established scale of intelligence, to that group of test questions which the child was able to answer correctly. The degree of intelligence of a child is estimated, accordingly, by the number of years by which its "age of intellectual development" differs from its actual age.

The method used in these examinations is a very simple one. First, it is determined which of the test questions corresponding to the child's real age have been perfectly answered. These form the basis. The examination then proceeds to groups of questions corresponding to higher ages. As a rule, only a part of these are answered correctly. This is continued no matter how far it may be necessary to go in the age scale of question groups, until we come to groups in which none of the questions is answered at all. The number of correct answers in those groups of test questions of which only part have been correctly answered is then summed up. Every five questions solved, no matter to how high an age they may correspond, are considered to mean one more year in the scale representing the age to which the intellectual development of the child corresponds.

If, for instance, a child six years old still solves all the tests devised for the seven-year-old children, then the basis for determining the child's age of intellectual development is seven years. If, now, the child is also able to solve three of the eight-year-old tests, one of the nine-year-old, and one of those for ten-year-old children, it must be considered to be equal in its intelligence to a child of eight.

Of course, only such tests may be used in the determination of intelligence which, on the one hand, have been selected so that, as far as possible, they may aim at "pure intelligence" and not at the store of information amassed by the aid of, and dependent on, chance circumstances, and which, on the other hand, are calculated accurately to follow the normal intellectual development of the child. It is true that the tests suggested by Binet and Simon,[1] which are widely used in measurements of intelligence, do not fulfil these requirements, for they include questions, the correct answers to which depend on knowledge acquired at school, and on external circumstances, such as the character of the surroundings in which the child lives. It has also been proved that the series of tests devised for the various degrees of age, especially those for younger children, are too easy. Probably this may partly be attributed to the fact that the tests were originally intended for working-class children.[2] However, although the system

[1] Binet et Simon, " Le développement de l'intelligence chez les enfants," *Année Psychologique*, vol. 14, 1908.

[2] Goddard has shown that of the seven-year-old children he has examined with the aid of the Binet-Simon series of tests, 58 per cent. were on the level of their age and 29 per cent. above that level. (Two thousand normal children measured by the Binet Measuring Scale of Intelligence, *Pedagog. Seminary*, vol. 18, p. 232 sqq.). According to Bobertag, " Über Intelligenzprüfung " (On the Examination of Intelligence), *Zeitschrift f. angewandte Psychologie*, vol. 6, p. 495 sqq., 44·5 per cent. of the seven- and eight-year-old children, and according to K. L. Johnstone, as many as 68 per cent. of the six- to seven-year-old children stood above the intelligence level of their age (quoted from Stern). Binet himself calculated the average difference in "intelligence age" between children of the upper and those of the lower classes to amount to about one and a half years. So this fact ought to be taken into account, when examining children of the upper classes. Investigations carried out by Ballard, Burt, Claparède, Descoudres, Goddard, Lipmann, Rossolimo, Spearman, W. Stern and his pupils, Terman, Thomson, Thorndike, Treves and Saffioti, Whipple, Yerkes, etc., also deal with this subject.

of tests proposed by Binet and Simon does not fulfil
all the requirements which we look upon as essential
in a test system which is to be universally applied,
nevertheless, thought it best, at the time, 1910, to
ascertain Erwin's degree of intelligence by means of
these tests, in order to be able to compare the results
of examinations carried out by other psychologists
with the results of my own researches. At that time
the revision of the Binet tests by Binet himself, and
by Bobertag, Goddard, Jaederholm, and Terman had
not yet been made, and those numerous new and skil-
fully devised mental tests which would certainly have
been much more appropriate for determining the intelligence and the degree of maturity of the child were not
yet available.

I began the experiments calculated to determine
Erwin's degree of intelligence with the tests devised for
seven-year-old children, Erwin's age at that time being
seven years. All these tests were solved correctly.[1]
There was only one test, the explanation and description
of a picture laid before the child—perhaps the best
test of all—which I did not employ, having regard to
the limits of the time then at my disposal ; I am of the
opinion, however, being aware of Erwin's admirable
talent for the description of things that had happened
to him, that he would undoubtedly have answered this
test also with great dexterity.

The tests for eight-year-old children were also all

[1] The following tests were made :—write down words spoken, count thirteen
pennies, tell the number of the ten fingers, repeat five figures heard, draw a
rhombus, drawn first by the examiner, recognize coins from a penny to a
crown, recognize missing parts in drawings.

C

answered correctly.[1] In fact Erwin, when answering these tests, did more than was to be expected from the average eight-year-old child, since he made no mistakes in spelling when writing the sentences dictated to him, and not only gave the names of the four chief colours, but also those of composite colours, and spontaneously added a remark on their light or dark character, and, finally, he quoted from a newspaper paragraph read to him not only the two items of information required by the tests, but in one case seven, in the other twelve extra items.

The tests of the series for nine-year-old children were also all answered correctly by Erwin.[2]

Out of the series for ten-year-old children he answered the following tests:—give the names of the months; form two sentences in which three given words occur; answer three easy questions designed to test general intelligence.[3] The test of recognizing coins was not answered, but this, in my opinion, is not a suitable test for the examination of intellectual capacity. Another test, the answering of five difficult questions,

[1] The tests were the following:—count backwards from twenty to one, state from memory the differences between two familiar objects, write to dictation, make the sum of seven pence (three pennies and two twopences), give the name of the four chief colours, and finally state two items of information from a newspaper paragraph read.

[2] These tests were the following:—define (concrete) objects by statements which go beyond the mere statement of what use is made of them; give eighty (Hungarian) pence in change for a crown; state six remembered facts; tell the days of the week; tell the date of to-day; put five weights in their proper succession.

[3] These questions were as follows: What ought one to do when one has missed a train? What ought one to do if one has broken an object which does not belong to one? What ought one to do if one goes to school and notices that it is later than usual?

Erwin was not able to solve correctly.[1] Finally I examined him by aid of the tests for eleven-year-old children. He answered two tests easily: to form a sentence from three words, and to name sixty words in three minutes; in fact, he enumerated seventy-seven words in three minutes instead of the number required. The test of criticizing sentences of absurd meaning he only answered partly, and in five questions he only succeeded with the first three.[2] In the last test of this series, to put a medley of words into logical order, he also partly succeeded, for he understood what the group of words was intended to mean, but was not able to convert them into a sentence. If we wish to act strictly according to the established method, these last tests should be omitted in estimating the degree of intelligence of a child; if, however, we take into account the extent to which he has succeeded in answering them, it may be right to count these two incompletely solved tests as one good point.

[1] The five difficult questions were the following : (1) What ought one to do if one has been struck by a friend by mistake? (2) What ought one to do, before undertaking something important? (3) Suppose some one asks your opinion on a person whom you know only slightly, what will you say? (4) Why is a wicked act, committed in anger, more excusable than a wicked act which is not committed in anger? (5) Why should a man be judged by his actions rather than by his words?

[2] The following absurd sentences were given :—(1) I have three brothers, Paul, Ernest and myself; can one say this? Why not? (2) Recently there was found in a forest a corpse, cut into eighteen pieces; some people thought that the case was one of suicide; is this possible? (3) Yesterday a cyclist had an accident on the road, which killed him; he was brought to a hospital from which they hope they will soon be able to dismiss him; is that possible? (4) I have just been reading in a newspaper about a railway accident, but it was not a serious one, only forty-eight people being killed; is this correct? (5) The other day a friend come to see me who complained that he was very badly off. He said he would kill himself some day, but not on a Friday, as this was an unlucky day for him; what do you think of this?

If, therefore, in determining Erwin's age of intellectual development, we take the ninth year as a basis, and take into account the three tests for ten-year-old children, and two tests for those of eleven, thus giving an additional total of five tests, which would be equivalent, according to Binet, to another year in the development of intelligence, the total difference by which Erwin's intelligence is in advance of normal children—this difference being expressed by the difference of the "age of intellectual development", and the real age—is three years. *Erwin is therefore in his general mental development at least three years in advance of his age.*

This is the result of the examination for general intelligence, using the first set of Binet-Simon tests as originally published in 1908. But the result remains the same, if we make use of the revised tests published after my experiments (1911). On the other hand, it must be remembered, when determining to what extent Erwin's intelligence is in advance of that of a normal child, that he cannot be considered a working-class child, but belongs, as far as the whole of his education is concerned, to the educated class. Yet even taking into account the difference between children of the educated and those of the working-class (this difference being, as we said before, equivalent to one year and a half; see note 2, on page 32), there still remains a space of at least one year and a half by which Erwin's intellectual ability in his seventh year of age was in advance of that of his coevals. If, however, we take the new scale of the Binet test system into account, which has been arrived at by adjusting the mental tests until the test series for every degree of age really corresponds to the normal capacity of children, Erwin's level of intelligence does not appear by any means in a less favourable light : on the contrary, it shows to advantage. According to Jaederholm's measurements [1] the child answered the tests for the seven- and eight-year-old children perfectly, also those for nine-year-old children, with the single exception of the criticism of absurdities (prescribed in Binet's system for children of eleven), which he only partly accomplished, giving three correct answers out of five. From among the tests devised for children ten years old, Erwin answered the first three correctly ; as to the last two, which have been added to the existing tests by the author, they were, of course, not used in this examination, but it is very likely that he would have been able to answer them correctly.[2]

It then became interesting to ascertain the extent to which Erwin's intelligence had continued to develop, and especially, whether, having passed his tenth year of age, he still possessed a greater intellectual capacity than that of other children of his age. It was found in April 1913 that Erwin could answer all the tests for ten-, eleven-, and twelve - year - old children embodied in Binet and Simon's original system drawn up in 1908.[3] The tests for children of eleven have

[1] G. A. Jaederholm, *Undersökningar över Intelligensmätningarnas*, Stockholm, 1914.

[2] The tests inserted were : Count backwards from forty-one, deducting three every time. How can one call cows, oxen, horses, sheep, etc. ? What are all these together?

[3] The Binet-Simon tests for thirteen-year-old children were insufficient.

already been mentioned on p. 35, those for twelve-year-old children, completed by a few subsidiary questions, were the following:—Describe and explain a picture, repeat seven figures, repeat a sentence of twenty-six syllables, find three rhymes in a minute, fill up words left out in a text, and, finally, a test of the child's power of grasping extraordinary situations. It should be mentioned here that Binet, later on, in 1911, modified his system of measurement,[1] and considerably reduced the requirements for children eleven and twelve years old; indeed, he recommended the tests for the eleven-year-old children to be used for those of twelve, and those for the twelve-year-old children for those of fifteen. We will leave it open whether these alterations are justified. Erwin answered all these questions and this proves that, at the age of ten, he still surpassed the boys of his age by *at least* two years and on the basis of the revised tests by even more, so that he might be considered equal to a normal child of thirteen to fourteen years of age.[2] About the

[1] Binet, "La mesure du developpement de l'intelligence chez les jeunes enfants," *Bull. de la soc. libre pour l'étude ps. de l'enfant*, Paris, 1911, Nos. 10, 11; Binet et Simon, "Nouvelles recherches sur la mesure du niveau intellectuel chez les enfants de l'école," *Année psychologique*, vol. 17, 1911.

[2] I have, besides those mentioned, made the following further experiments with Erwin:—(1) Give the even numbers from thirty to two backwards. Erwin required 16 seconds in which to do this (1911). Comparative experiments with lower-class children have shown that, out of ten children of the same age, nine solved this test without a mistake in an average time of 29·4 seconds (the shortest time taken was 13 seconds, the longest 48 seconds). (2) Give the uneven numbers from twenty-nine to one backwards. It took 13·5 seconds (1911). This task was accomplished without a mistake by only one child (in 1 min. 15 seconds), with mistakes by three (in an average time of 34 seconds), the other six not being able to solve it at all. (3) Repeat series of figures given orally. A series composed of five figures, presented in the rhythm three-two, and one composed of six figures in the rhythm three-

tests for eleven-year-old children only so much can be said, with reference to Erwin, that he was able to solve two of those which occurred in the Binet tests; as to what result would have been attained with the three other tests which were not employed, nothing can be said. As an aggregate result, we may safely state, however, that the degree of maturity of Erwin *according to the Jaederholm system of tests* corresponded to that of a *child of ten years of age.*

If we wish to determine Erwin's "intelligence age" according to Terman's mental test system,[1] we may quote the following results: The tests for children seven and eight years of age were perfectly answered by Erwin. Terman's subsidiary questions could not, of course, be checked, but there is no reason to suppose

three was repeated by Erwin correctly; another series consisting of seven figures, presented in the rhythm four-three or three-three-one, he was not able to reproduce without mistakes (1911). After the lapse of one year, Erwin's memory for figures developed to such an extent that he was able to repeat, without mistakes and without halting, a series consisting of seven units given in the rhythm three-three-one, one consisting of eight units given in the rhythm three-three-two, and one of nine units in the rhythm three-three-three (1912). In the course of comparative experiments ten children were able to reproduce the series of five figures correctly, only nine could reproduce that of six figures, and only one that of seven figures. Among ten children eleven years old (which, therefore, were from two-three years older than Erwin) only three could repeat the seven-figure, two the eight-figure and only one the nine-figure series. (4) In order to find how far "visual counting," i.e. the grasping of numerical relations of an entirely visual character was developed in Erwin, I put before the child, according to the method of Katz and Révész, twelve counters of the same colour, and asked him to remove from the series every second, then every third one, and so on. He solved the problem successfully as far as removing every fifth mark. When I tried to make the task more difficult by using counters of different colours, instead of those of the same colour, he still succeeded in solving the problem without any difficulty (1911). Compare with this: D. Katz and G. Révész, "Experimentell-psychologische Untersuchungen an Hühnern," *Zeitschrift f. Psychologie,* vol. 50, pp. 93-116, 1908.

[1] Terman, L. M., Stanford Revision I. *Source Material* II. *Guide.*

that Erwin could not have answered them; on the contrary, we have every reason to believe that he would have done so correctly.[1] Four of the tests for nine-year-old children were solved correctly; those which consisted of reading four figures backwards and making rhymes were not tried.

Of the two subsidiary questions the first was answered correctly and the second would probably not have caused Erwin any difficulty.[2]

Of the six fundamental and the three subsidiary questions for ten-year-old children, four tests were answered successfully, one (absurdities) partly, and the last one was not answered. As there were two more correct answers to tests belonging to the test series for twelve-year-old children, we may assert with safety that *according to Terman's system of intellectual measurement also,* Erwin had preceded his age by *at least three years.*[3]

These, then, are the results which I obtained by the use of this well-established form of measurement. But this method was not sufficient in the case of Erwin. It is useful for showing us the discrepancy

[1] Subsidiary tests for seven-year-old children: Give the days of the week and repeat three figures in inverse order. For children eight years old: Recognition of six coins (a test about which I have already expressed my opinion) and writing to dictation, of which ability the child has often given sufficient proof.

[2] Give the names of the months and the aggregate value of two stamps.

[3] If we compare results by the aid of the revised Binet test system effected by Bobertag, we get perhaps a still better result, since Erwin solved four out of the eight tests intended for children of the age of eleven perfectly well, one in its greater part well, there being only one which he was unable to answer; the remaining two not having been applied to him. According to this system, the level of his intelligence corresponds, at least, to that of a child between ten and eleven years old. Bobertag, "Über Intelligenzprüfungen nach der Methode Binet-Simon," *Zeitschr. für angewandte Psychologie,* vols. 5, 6, 1911.

between a child's age and the degree of its intelligence, and it may be used for establishing an order of sequence, as regards intelligence, between children of the same age, but the method is too theoretical, it merely sheds light on certain aspects of the intelligence, and it is only satisfactory in the case of examinations *en masse*, in which individual differences may be neglected with impunity. But when it is precisely these that are essential, in cases where we wish to arrive clearly at those features of the child's intelligence which are particularly developed—and this holds good, especially in the case of highly-gifted children—this method is unsatisfactory.

In our case the inadequacy of this measurement of intelligence by tests is proved in a most striking manner. We get a most indistinct impression of Erwin, one which is in noway characteristic of him, if we base our conclusions merely on these tests of intelligence, for precisely that quality which is most remarkable in his intellect, its brilliance, is not exposed by this method. It is certainly not due to prejudice on my part that I consider Erwin's intelligence to be beyond comparison with that of normally developed children.

I observed that Erwin, as soon as he had acquired the knowledge necessary for certain intellectual operations, was generally able to perform them. This was particularly noticeable in the case of tasks connected with music. The degree of certainty with which he expressed his judgments on difficult questions, and the deep truths that lay in his utterances were almost incredible. He analysed his own inner life in the manner of a trained psychologist, he talked about his observations on himself clearly and consistently, and that which will appear still more marvellous to many people—he expressed himself with great caution and in remarkably pregnant phraseology. He often asked me whether what he was about to tell me would get "into the book," for in this case, he said, "I want to express myself correctly, and you must pay great attention to me; for a single wrongly-chosen word may alter the meaning of the whole thing." It was also characteristic of him to search eagerly at times for the right expressions and, if words failed him, to convey his meaning by expressive gestures. In the end, he made everything clear, sometimes repeated what he had said, and then asked whether one had understood it correctly. It is really no exaggeration when I say that what he told me about music was more interesting and approached more nearly to the truth, than that which I have heard from many musicians. Indeed, musicians, like most artists, are hardly ever able to describe their own experiences, especially when alluding to those processes of consciousness which move them during creative activity and interpretation. They generally express themselves ambiguously and with conventional and not very expressive gestures. Most of them, indeed, do not like to be asked questions, they easily get confused, and, sometimes, do not even know precisely what one wants of them, and, as a result, their answers are obscure.

It is quite different in the case of Erwin. He grasps the questions with absolute precision ; it is not even necessary to formulate them in any particular way, or to adapt them at all to his age. It is possible to talk to him as to any grown-up person, and one derives quite as much pleasure from it !

I will now corroborate my statements by a few examples, which, however, naturally give only a faint idea of the manner in which Erwin's genius manifests itself in personal intercourse.

As he showed great love of nature, I often asked him, that spring, to take a walk with me. On a beautiful clear spring day, when he was overwhelmed by its beauty, we discussed the marvellous and affecting character of nature. I talked about forests and mountains, and from these he passed on to modern painting. He said that, although modern painters use beautiful, vivid colours, yet these colours do not even approach in beauty the colours of nature. He spoke of a picture which he had seen in the house of a family of his acquaintance, in which the sky was painted green. He found the picture and the colours very pretty, because they were effective, but he expressed the view that painters ought not to paint in a manner so opposed to nature. He added, in quite a naïve way, that the painter might paint the sky green, if he found this pretty, but he must not make it absolutely green, but ought to use a bluish-green tint. When I thereupon suggested to him that, perhaps, he meant to imply that the object of painting was to produce a faithful reproduction of nature, he answered suddenly that he did not believe that "a painter should paint things exactly as he sees them in nature, for this would be impossible, but at least he ought not to paint against nature. This painter wanted to paint something beautiful *purposely*" (the word "purposely" was strongly accentuated), "but that was only a picturesque affectation.[1] I love nature best," he continued, "the colours of nature, such, for instance, as the beautiful grey and brown of this tree-trunk. It is so splendid when the sun shines through the branches of the trees, and when nature seems so alive, for nature lives also, and it is this that I express by music."

To the question whether he expressed the sunshine, the songs of the birds, etc. in his compositions, he replied : "Not that, but the emotion, which is awakened in me by the beautiful forest. The joy of living, the life of nature, the joy which nature gives me, which is within me. . . . I do not like", he continued, "to compose sad things, for I do not like sadness, I only love the joy of living." At the word "joy of living," which he uttered often and in a most expressive way, he stretched out both his arms, as if he wanted to embrace the whole beauty of nature.

To my question whether, during composition, he ever thought of people, or of certain occurrences of his life, he replied that that happened sometimes as, for instance, in the case of his *Ballad*, but, in most cases,

[1] That Erwin here reproaches the painter with his *purpose* of painting in a certain way corresponds to his view that it is only possible to compose a musical piece when the composition is born "spontaneously," and not of a preconceived purpose.

nothing of the sort came into his mind. "Thus, for
instance", he said, "I thought of nothing when composing the *Romance;* it is just like somebody who sings
for his own pleasure, he has no other intention, but just
to sing."

Later, I asked him whether during the whole time he
worked at a piece he kept up the same state of feeling.
He replied to this, that he did so, indeed, as far as
possible, and then continued : "When composing,
one must not always give way to one's *heart*, the head
must also be consulted. Often it is necessary that the
heart should be silenced, pushed into the background,
otherwise the composition will become weak.[1]

"In composing, one wants the heart and the head ;
the heart alone or the head alone is not sufficient, for
the heart may turn away a man from what is genuine
music, and the head alone does not produce an expression of emotion, but merely scientific music, which
may be interesting, but is not always beautiful. But
one must not allow oneself to be led astray by emotion,
for, if emotion alone rules, one does not produce a
composition, or rather, one does produce a composition,
but it is not a success ; it is not so fine, so well worked-
out, as it ought to be."

It was difficult for Erwin to express himself when I
asked him whether in every composition a separate
emotional idea ought to be expressed. "No," he
remarked, "there are also compositions in which one
finds none." The lack of an emotional idea in a piece

---

[1] "Weak" was probably not intended to mean "of inferior value", but
means simply "lacking in strength".

he characterized by the following remarkable comparison : "In such a case my composition looks like people walking on the road, tram-cars running, children whistling on the street; it means nothing, only music."

When I asked him whether he was able to compose when in a sad state of mind, he replied : "No, in a such state of mind I cannot compose either a sad or a joyful piece. When I am composing something melancholy, I am not quite so gay as I am now. If I am very gay, I can neither put melancholy tunes into notes, nor can I perform a melancholy piece of music."

We now began to talk about the interpretation of other people's compositions. In the course of the conversation I asked him whether, when performing a piece, he believed he was in the same state of emotion as the composer when he created the piece. He replied that he did not know whether his state of emotion was the same as that of the composer, he just played the piece as he understood it to be meant, "as it accords with my *beauty of emotion*.[1] How I play a certain piece depends on my state of emotion ; if I am able to bring my own state of emotion well into the piece, it goes well, if not, it is not a success. In reproduction, it is possible that the piece may have as much influence on one's emotion as one's emotion has on the way one performs the piece."

On another occasion, we talked about composers, and I asked Erwin to characterize some of them.

---

[1] In the Hungarian language, such an expression does not exist ; he created it himself.

Erwin began with J. S. Bach, of whose works
at that time he knew only his *Inventions* in two and
more parts. "Bach was the composer", he said,
"who brought music to perfection. Everything which
he composed is *solid, concise, and briefly expressed.*
Bach is the stem of music, he stands on the highest
summit of music, but not on the summit of emotion.
In his works only the *music* is perfect, but not the
emotional idea."

Erwin makes, as we see here, a sharp distinction
between the emotional substance and the purely musical
substance of a work. When, for instance, he says:
"I am now going to talk about Bach as a composer,"
he means by this that he intends to talk only of the
formal and purely musical side of his compositions.
He once expressed himself in a very happy manner,
when he said: "As opposed to the emotional idea
expressed, stand the forms, the harmonies, the part-
writing, and the grandeur of a work: it is possible to
compose in a very beautiful and interesting manner
without expressing beautiful or rich emotion."

He continued: "Bach was solid and austere in his
music. Beethoven lowered the standard of perfection
of *music* a little, for, besides his musical sense, he
already had a strong sense of emotion. Of course,
Bach did not lack the sense of emotion entirely; only
in him it was small compared with his enormous sense
of music.

"Schumann lowered the standard of solidity set by
Bach still more. As a painter of emotional conditions
he is finer than as a composer; to him the emotional

state to be expressed was much more important than music.[1] His music is *quite simple and elaborate*. That is to say, all his music, especially his part-writing, appears incredibly elaborate, and, yet, it is when one looks at the notes surprisingly simple. To the ear, Schumann's music is delicate and complicated, to the eye, on the other hand, very simple. It is in this that the greatness of Schumann lies, that he was able to produce such intricate music by such simple means. But it is not sufficient to be simple, for that does not necessarily mean beauty of emotion. Take, for instance, a C major chord. One ought to compose in a simple manner, which, however, should at the same time be beautiful. The emotions expressed by Schumann were always simple ones, and of such a character that it was possible to express them beautifully in music." I then asked Erwin to say something about Mozart and to compare him with whichever other composer stands nearest to him. Erwin had already, a few years before, expressed his view that Mozart and Beethoven were the greatest composers, although of Mozart's works he only knew the sonatas for the piano, and even at the time of uttering the following remarks he did not know many of his works beside these, a circumstance that should not for a moment be left out of consideration when estimating the value of the ensuing criticisms. If we keep this in mind, it is not surprising that, of the whole variety of Mozart's genius,

[1] I presume that Erwin does not here oppose emotional to musical expression, but that the contrast meant is that between the state of feeling expressed in music and all the purely formal elements of expression.

Erwin should have recognized only the one side. For if we do not know his operas and his chamber music many, indeed the most essential, traits are lacking from our impression of Mozart.

"Mozart stands much farther off from Bach than he does from Beethoven; he is related to Bach only in so far as they were both classical composers. To Beethoven, Mozart stands in much closer relation, for Beethoven's music was not so solid and austere, it was not *music only*, as Bach's was. Mozart was more delicate and light in feeling than Beethoven, but he was not so subtle in music and in his part-writing. Beethoven wrote more serious music than Mozart, for he probably experienced much more sorrow and bitterness than Mozart, and that is why Beethoven's melodies speak to one's heart more than Mozart's. Mozart was a much more joyful person, and that is shown in his music. I, personally, care more for joyful music, but nevertheless I like Beethoven better than Mozart. But I know so few of Mozart's works that I cannot say anything certain about him."

About Brahms, of whose works Erwin at that time knew only a few pieces for the piano (intermezzos, rhapsodies) he did not wish to express an opinion. But when I urged him to do so, he said that Brahms, as far as he was able to judge him from those of his works with which he was familiar, was not a *romantic*, as is generally supposed, but a classical composer, although not an "old classical" but a "new classical" one.

About Grieg, Erwin made the following remarks:

D

"Grieg is a monotonous, sonorous composer, he expresses gloomy emotions; this is the effect of the North. He has written several wonderfully fine pieces, with very beautiful harmonies, which however recur too often. He was not able to picture feelings in all his compositions; namely, wherever he is monotonous, he is also lacking in emotion." Then Erwin suddenly paused, reflected for some time intently, and continued as follows: "Indeed, it is possible that his monotonous compositions express just as richly-varied emotions as are expressed for us by the works of Schumann. For there, up in the North, there must be other kinds of natural harmonies than here in our part of the world; it is true, of course, that music remains music everywhere, in our part of the world as well as in the North or in Argentina; but the moods of nature may have another effect on a Northern man than on us, for our feelings are different from theirs; in spite of this, however, I do not mean to say that they are not the same kind of people as we are; they are exactly the same human beings, they have exactly the same 'organization', but music arouses other kinds of feelings in them. There they don't say of Grieg's music that it is monotonous, but we say so."

These words, of course, undoubtedly show traces of what Erwin had heard about Grieg, but he said everything in so well-considered a manner and was so obviously reflecting on it, that I had the impression that he had thought out what he had heard, and made it his own.

When I asked Erwin to say something about Richard Wagner, he showed great joy, became a little

excited, and said that he was able to tell me a great
deal about Wagner. He brought a chair, and sat
down opposite to me, and after remarking that, properly
speaking, his opinion about Wagner was not yet a
fixed one, as he knew too few of his works, he began :
" I shall first speak of Wagner as a composer. Wagner
was a very fine part-writer and a composer of great
verve. I cannot say that he always made *beautiful*
harmonies, but his harmonies always sound *full* and
sonorous. His compositions are never empty or un-
interesting, for whenever there is a want of melody
he makes up for it by filling his pieces with something
else, for instance, with harmonies; and, if they are empty
in one sense, they are full and great in another. As
a portrayer of feeling Wagner is very strong, although,
among composers, the one to whom he bears the
strongest resemblance is Bach. But he had more
feeling than Bach and was more highly cultured ; still,
as regards fullness and strength, his music stands
nearest to that of Bach. Wagner was, at the same
time, a classical and a romantic composer. He was
classical as regards the grandeur of his works ; but, on
the other hand, he was a romantic composer as far
as the emotions he expressed were concerned."

Erwin now wished to speak about a modern composer of operas. When he asked me to name one, I
suggested Bizet, for I knew that among composers of
operas, Bizet was his favourite.

" Bizet has composed very serious melodies, but by
this I do not mean that his melodies are gloomy or too
serious, but that they are well-thought-out and carefully

considered. Of Schumann, one might say the same thing, but while his melodies are of a pleasantly serious, and dreamy character, Bizet's are rather dramatic. Bizet's harmony is marvellous." (He gave a few examples.) "His music is always beautiful and interesting; whatever is lacking in one direction is made up for in another, just as with Wagner, but Bizet has not written with such fullness and strength as Wagner.

"Bizet has composed more serious music than Verdi —Verdi on the other hand has more inventive genius and is more melodious than Bizet. Thus, for instance, in the first act of *Traviata* we find nothing but *arias;* there is no break when the tunes cease and something else comes in their place." (He produced the vocal score of *Traviata* and proved this.) "The opposite occurs with Wagner. In his works you find recitatives; from a musical point of view, there is much grandeur in this, and it is very interesting, but when a layman hears it, he says 'Oh, how tedious this is!' Besides, Bizet's melodies have a greater value than those of Verdi. Verdi's melodies all came from his heart; he wrote them down exactly as they occurred to him and altered nothing in them. Bizet on the other hand reflected first, whether he could not express something better in this or that manner, and thus he created, though often at the cost of melody, works which were musically better and nobler."

About quite modern composers Erwin did not wish to speak; he does not like them very much, and for that reason he did not want to express any opinion about them. I asked him whether, perhaps, he could say something about Puccini. "All right, about Puccini, the fellow with the fifths, I can say something," he said, and laughed heartily as he spoke. "Puccini is something of a Bohemian. I do not say this because he has composed works like *La Bohème* (after all, Leoncavallo did this too), but he really gives me this impression. Whenever Puccini shows invention, it is always very beautiful, rich and wonderful, but when melody is lacking I always have an impression that he is saying: 'Now let us go on the spree'. I hope he won't challenge me to a duel for saying so.[1] It is not in music that Puccini becomes frivolous, but in his expression of emotion (first act of *Butterfly* : 'Amore o grillo'). And the fifths, after all, begin to pall on one in the end. If the consecutive fifths were at least musically beautiful, all would be well, but they are only so to a very small extent. Also they do not come from the heart.

"Of Mascagni I can say less indeed, but nicer things. His melodies are wonderful and deeply-felt, much more natural than those of Puccini, for in the case of Puccini they are often made *purposely*, but with Mascagni this never occurs. His harmonies also are very beautiful and simple ; he does not make use of everything that is forbidden by Richter and Rischbieter,"[2] he added, laughing.

The following statement made by him not long ago

[1] Erwin knows Puccini personally and is on very good terms with him.
[2] Two well-known teachers of the theory of harmony.

is specially characteristic of the relation in which he stood at that time to modern composers, and also of the self-conscious, critical and well-considered manner in which he dealt with musical questions, and the foresight with which he endeavoured to control his own future development.

"Some days ago I played through a few operas by Puccini, and found wonderful melodies in them, which I performed with great pleasure. I like Puccini particularly, his melodies speak to my heart, and I cannot withstand the effect he has upon me. But they only please my heart, not my head. As his music, quite against my will, has so strong an effect on me—for I know quite well that it only acts upon my emotions, and that is not enough—I fear that if I continue to play this music of Puccini, which gives me so much pleasure, I shall gradually come under his influence and compose in a manner similar to his. And I do not want this to happen. That is why I suddenly put away the score and set myself to playing the most *simple* and easy pieces of Schumann (Album for the Young). Then I perceived how different, how deep and simple everything is in Schumann, and that I must learn from him."

How largely these reflections may be the result of what he had heard from others I am not in a position to ascertain; but it is amazing with what assurance and conviction he gave voice to them, how he marshalled his thoughts, how he developed one thought from another, and how, in conversation, he argued with himself, and tried to refute objections which presented themselves (see Grieg). The fact that he reflected for a considerable time, and created quite original phrases in the course of formulating his opinions, proves that his judgments were the result of mature reflection, and in the nature of a personal experience.

Evidently only a part of his very independent judgments were the result of reflections on opinions he had heard ; most of his utterances their very substance stamps with the mark of originality. To this must be added his general behaviour during these discussions.

He expresses all his opinions with assurance, and with the confidence of a thinker whose judgment is based on mature reflection ; he does not say anything rashly, he is very cautious, he does not jump to conclusions, and if any judgment appears to him too sweeping, he qualifies it later. Wherever he is afraid he has not expressed himself quite clearly, he offers a subsequent explanation. Questioned at different times, he always remains consistent, and does not allow himself to be disconcerted by the different opinions of other people. When reflecting and comparing, he is always prepared with finished propositions concerning the different composers.

He never remains content with a general superficial valuation, such as we find in people who are weak in their critical faculty ; on the contrary, he always goes into details. These details are invariably the *essential* ones ; he never speaks about things of secondary importance, a fact that would be difficult to explain if he only reproduced things which he had heard.

His remarks are sometimes quite original, occasionally surprising (his opinion on Schumann and on Wagner); but even when he consents to adopt the general view, he expresses himself in an original, simple, and childlike manner, and says things which grown-up people would avoid for fear of appearing trivial.

I have emphasized a few of his characteristics; but even without these indications the attentive reader will find sufficiently distinct proofs of originality.

We may now put the question whether, in view of the evidence we have collected, we may consider Erwin a precocious child. The answer to this question evidently depends on our definition of precocity. If we mean by a precocious child one that soon discovers the field most particularly adapted to his gifts, and acquires, at an early age, greater knowledge and ability in this field than his contemporaries, we must, of course, consider Erwin, and any other children who exhibit remarkable intellectual or technical superiority over others of the same age, as precocious. But I do not approve of this definition. I should not call children of this description precocious, but simply *possessed of special faculties showing themselves at an early age.* It is not possible, for instance, to say of all great musicians and artists, whose artistic gifts have been prematurely awakened, that they have been, as children, precocious —this would not correspond with the image we evoke when we employ the word " precocious ".

It is just as much beside the mark to speak of precocity in the case of a child like Erwin, whose

general mental faculties have preceded his age by a
few years, and who merely responds to tests ordinarily
applied only to older children.   Such a child is *predeveloped*, but not precocious.

We will use the expression "precocious" only
concerning a child who, not only with regard to his
intellectual aspect but *according to the whole scope of his
mental life*, may be placed on an equality with one
much older; who, in his whole view of life, resembles
a grown-up person, and uses his experience and the
knowledge he possesses in practical life in a way similar
to that of adult people.   In such a child the original,
naïve confidence is lacking, he is not straightforward,
he thinks little of infantile things, and endeavours to
place himself in the battle-line and take up a definite
position in life.   *In a precocious child the child element
is lacking.*   Neither is he a real adult, he is not
developed naturally, he lacks the progressive, undisturbed life of the bud, even as he lacks the real
experience of life possessed by grown-up people.   A
precocious child need not be gifted; for, even if his
feats of intelligence are equal to those of older children,
they lose their character and their significance as signs
of talent, and he fails to reach the intellectual level
which, judging by the intellectual qualities we have
mentioned, might rightly be expected of him.

Erwin was a child in the full sense of the word;
a clever, gay, friendly, charming boy.   After overcoming the first shyness, which he always cast off
quickly, he became friendly, confident and amiable;
and he charmed every one with whom he spent any

length of time. He was intrinsically honest and open-hearted, and he always said frankly what he meant. He was ready in his answers, and his replies were always clever, reasonable, and witty. He teased one with endless questions, which it was necessary to answer, whether it were possible or not. He played as children play, was fond of boyish exploits, and enjoyed them very much.

Only on superficial observation, when biased by the knowledge that one was speaking to a composer, did one gain a first impression that his mode of expression and will-power were those of an older child. A more thorough observation of the trend of his mind and soul showed, however, that his activities, if they were in any way more developed than those of his contemporaries, were so only in so far as they were connected with his artistic activity. That the activity of his feelings, and more especially his strength of will, were, in every respect, more prominent than in other children of his age, was by no means the case. This does not exclude the fact that his will-power was capable of great achievements where musical work was concerned.

He often sat for hours at the piano or at his desk, when he wished to transcribe his compositions. At the time that he composed his *Ballad*, he could only write very indistinctly, and a rather unmusical singing-master wrote down the piece for him as he dictated it. The child sat at the piano, and, owing to the inefficiency of the teacher, he had to play the bars separately to him several times, besides having to correct the manuscript.

This was very tedious work, and I was astonished that a little child—he was hardly six years of age at the time—could show so strong a will and so keen an enthusiasm.   Later, when he wrote down his compositions himself, his will-power and patience were not less admirable.

But, if we consider the matter more closely and seek an adequate reason for these remarkable feats of endurance we find that there is little essential difference between this exercise of will-power and the normal impulse towards activity of children, which finds its most distinct expression in the various games they play.   The admirable patience and concentration exhibited by children when tearing up paper, dismembering flowers, taking mechanisms to pieces, building with wooden bricks, and playing various games of patience, correspond quite well with Erwin's behaviour in composing.   When composing, Erwin experiences all the pleasure a child feels when playing ; the achieving of something, the solving of difficulties, the carrying out of some work : he does not look upon composing as a duty, a cumbersome piece of work, but it causes him an enjoyment similar to that found in the plastic or pictorial games of imitation (as, for instance, drawing or modelling), or other creative games of children.   It is thus seen that, in spite of his great will-power, it is not necessary to look upon this side of his psychic life as predeveloped.

NOTE

It will perhaps interest many people if I here give an account of Erwin's feats of draughtsmanship, which may well serve as an argument for the fact that he may not be considered as predeveloped as regards all the

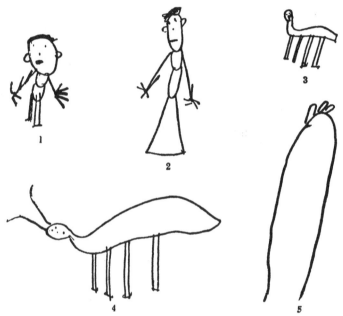

PLATE I.—Drawings made in 1910. Spontaneous Drawings.

utterances of the infantile soul. Indeed it seems as though ·his achievements in this respect remained below those of less gifted children.[1] In particular, the pictures drawn in 1913 seem to prove this (see

[1] Compare : E. Barnes, "A Study on Children's Drawings," *Pedagogical Seminary*, 1893; H. T. Lukens, "A Study on Children's Drawings in the Early Years," *Ped. Seminary*, 1896; S. Levinstein, *Kinderzeichnungen bis zum 14. Lebensjahr*, Leipzig, 1905.

Plate IV).   It is also both instructive and amusing
to put the drawings and the compositions side by side
and observe the enormous contrast !

On Plate I, I show first, five spontaneous drawings
of his.   The subjects depicted were : 1, a man ; 2, a
woman ; 3, a dog ; 4, a cow ; 5, a tree.   The drawings
in Plate II were copies from drawings.   These were :

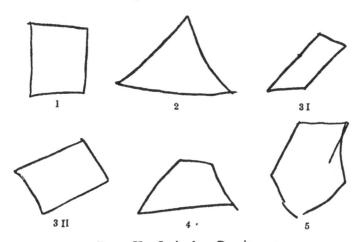

PLATE II.—Copies from Drawings.

1, a square ; 2, a triangle ; 3, a rhombus ; 4, a tra-
pezium ; 5, a hexagon.   Plate III contains drawings
made from *models*.   The following objects were given :
1, a table ; 2, a chair ; 3, a cube ; 4, a cylinder of
cardboard.   Finally Plate IV gives an idea of Erwin's
draughtsmanship some years later.   Figure 1 is said
to be a striking portrait ; 2, a silk hat ; 3, a table ; and
4, a cube, drawn from models.   The drawings in the
first three Plates were made when he was eight years
old, those of the fourth Plate when he was eleven.

What is most characteristic in such drawings of children has been expressed by Katz in the following sentence: "The child does not reproduce what he

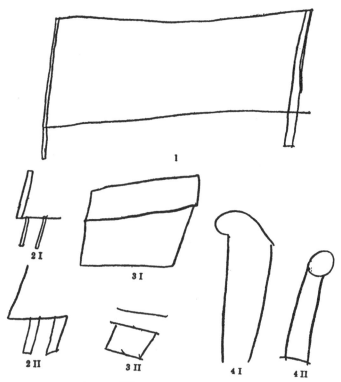

PLATE III.—Drawings after Models.

perceives, but rather what he knows about objects perceived." This peculiarity of infantile draughtsmanship, *viz.* that the child in his drawings illustrates his own knowledge about things, is already apparent in drawings of objects of two dimensions, and is seen still more clearly in drawings representing objects of three

dimensions. As good examples, the cow (Plate I), the
table and the silk hat (Plate IV) may be quoted ; also
a house in which, as well as the house front, the
cellars are portrayed (not reproduced), and the table
(Plate III) which is drawn with two legs only, but in
which, on the other hand, the objective proportions of
the flat top are strongly accentuated, while the per-
spective is altogether neglected.   In the drawings 3 and
4 of Plate III, a compromise was effected between the

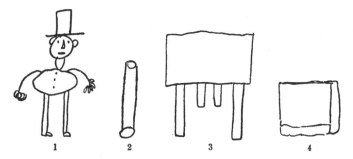

PLATE IV.—Drawings made in 1913.

child's knowledge of objects (i.e. of what he believes
actually exists in the object) and what he saw
directly.   In the case of the cube I the objective proportions of the dimensions and the objective position
of the lid were observed.   In the case of cube II the
perceptual content was exceeded to an even greater
degree, for the upper plane is simply alluded to by a
parallel line.   In depicting the cylinder, the knowledge that the top is of circular form is expressed
by a circle ; the complex of actual perception, on the
other hand, is expressed by the fact that Erwin has only
drawn one circle and a sharply cut-off base line.   The

last drawing seems to show that Erwin's work, in contrast to Katz's draughtsman, is based more on naïve experience and on immediate perception than on objective qualities, and that he is more influenced by appearance than by knowledge, which is well in accordance with his nature as an artist.

6. Investigation of Elementary Acoustic and Musical Faculties

WE now arrive at the essential part of our inquiry, the analysis of Erwin's *musical and acoustic faculties*. I have endeavoured, as far as possible, to test these capacities by making use of a series of experiments, in order to be able to record numerical results, which it is practically impossible to do when one confines oneself to mere observation.[1] One of the reasons which lead me to consider it particularly advisable to adopt this method is because I hope that later, when similar cases have been investigated in a like manner, scientists may arrive at some interesting conclusions, the result of comparative research concerning the abilities of highly-gifted young musicians—a branch of investigation that is indispensable for the foundation of certain general principles, and in determining the factors which have a decisive influence on artistic development.

[1] This investigation led me later on to establish tests for the examination of musical capacity, which are equally applicable to the case of those trained in music as to others, and to adults as well as to children. I also gave particular attention to the task of effecting a *quantitative* determination of the capacity for music; for particulars see " Prüfung der Musikalität ", *Zeitschrift f. Psychologie*, vol. 85, 1920, p. 163 seq. Comp. C. E. Seashore, *The Psychology of Musical Talent*, Boston, 1919, and a few other investigations on this subject carried out by the psychological laboratory of the University of Iowa, *Psychological Monographs*, vol. 31, 1922.

PERFECT PITCH

At my very first interview with Erwin I discovered that he possessed "perfect pitch." He was able instantly to state the musical name of any note or chord played upon the piano. He was also able to sing any desired note at command. To exclude the possibility of his making use of an interval during the work on perfect pitch, I took care to separate the various notes sounded by pauses, or by interposing between them sound-combinations devoid of meaning.

Erwin's sense of absolute pitch is based on the *recognition of tone-qualities*[1]—such, indeed, is almost always the case with the more finely-developed forms of perfect pitch. His decisions as to what note had been sounded were, as a rule, uttered very quickly, without reflection, and expressed with a feeling of absolute certainty. Erwin usually named the note played to him immediately, and, when judging very high or very low notes, never, as far as I could observe, made use of the device of transposing them vocally into the more familiar middle register.

It is a well-known fact that the sense of absolute pitch is developed to a very different degree in different persons. In the first place, it is generally admitted that differences exist as to the range of sounds covered by perfect pitch. Thus we meet people whose gift extends over almost the whole range of the musical register ; this

---

[1] Révész, G., *Grundlegung der Tonpsychologie*, 1913, p. 100. By *tone-quality* I understand that quality of sounds which returns after regular intervals of one octave and is indicated by the names *c*, *d*, *e*, etc. By *pitch*, on the other hand, I mean that which is continually changing with the changing vibrations and which is expressed by the position of the octaves.

I call complete *absolute pitch*. Then we see cases in which the sense is only perfect with regard to sounds within a part of the musical register ; we might give to a faculty limited in this way the name of *regional absolute pitch*.[1]

I have been able to ascertain that Erwin's sense of absolute pitch is complete, and that it extends over so wide a range that it has probably never been surpassed.

In order to be able to compare Erwin's capacity in this direction with that of other people, I tested him, in a series of experiments, with the identical notes and on the same instrument (piano) as Stumpf used in his experiments on perfect pitch.[2] The notes were taken from the regions C_1 to B_1, a to g^1 sharp and g^3 to f^4 sharp. The total number of notes given, in my experiments, were thirteen in each region.

The result was that, with low notes, between C_1 and B_1 eleven correct answers were given out of thirteen, with middle notes, between a and g^1 sharp, thirteen correct answers out of thirteen, and with high notes, between g^3 and f^4 sharp, thirteen out of thirteen.

The most favourable sets of experiments among those made by Stumpf with excellent musicians furnish the following proportion of correct answers :

	Low notes		*Middle notes*		*High notes*	
Popper	10 out of 13		13 out of 13		12 out of 13	
Stumpf	8	,, 13	13	,, 13	6	,, 13
Schenkl	2	,, 8	8	,, 10	6	,, 12
Sladek	3	,, 7	6	,, 10	2	,, 13
Nyiregyházi	11	,, 13	13	,, 13	13	,, 13

[1] Comp. Révész, G., *Grundlegung der Tonpsychologie*, p. 100.

[2] Stumpf, C., *Tonpsychologie*, Vol. I, 1883, p. 310, and Vol. II, 1890, p. 369.

Erwin, as may be seen, has, therefore, supplied more correct answers than the persons examined by Stumpf. O. Abraham, an investigator whose name is well-known in scientific literature on account of his sense of absolute pitch, has probably also been surpassed by Erwin, since in the region between C_1 and B_1 Abraham did not give such good results as Erwin; indeed, in this region, between thirty and eighty per cent. of his answers were incorrect.

In order to obtain a more exact impression of the precision of Erwin's gift, and, more especially to ascertain the extent of the perfection of his musical ear, I made him adjust a "Sound Variator" (Stern's system),[1] so as to emit notes of a given *quality* and *pitch*. Although the child did not pay particular attention to these experiments, which were of a kind that naturally did not strike his fancy, the adjustments he made were very satisfactory.

> When a^1 was asked for, the apparatus was adjusted to emit a note of 448 vibrations.
>
> When a^2 was asked for, the apparatus was adjusted to emit a note of 895 vibrations.
>
> When e^1 was asked for, the apparatus was adjusted to emit a note of 333 vibrations.
>
> When f^2 was asked for, the apparatus was adjusted to emit a note of 982 vibrations.

It is noteworthy that, in these experiments, the number of vibrations corresponding to the sounds asked

---

[1] Apparatus for producing a continuous series of sounds. Comp. E. B. Titchener, *A Text-book of Psychology*, 1919, p. 100.

for, do not appear to coincide with international pitch.
But these experiments were not made in my own laboratory, and I had, to my regret, no opportunity to verify
the tuning of the pipes.   It must also be taken into
consideration that the tuning of pianos does not always
correspond to international pitch ; and that as the names
of the notes, in this case, are associated with *heard*
sounds, they would probably not correspond exactly
with the international scale of tuning.   But this is of
no importance as regards our experiment ; what interests
us is merely the degree of exactitude with which Erwin
adjusted the absolute pitches.   The capacity for adjust-
ment, and with it, the degree of fineness of perfect pitch
is only determined by the amount of inaccuracy in the
adjustments.   This indeed was very slight in the case
of Erwin, especially if we take into account his youth
and lack of practice, as the average deviation with $n = 10$,
is only $\pm$ 1 vibration at a_1, $\pm$ 5 vibrations at a_2 and $\pm$ 2
at e_1.   A guarantee of the correctness of the adjustments
is also to be found in the fact that the notes, as adjusted,
stand to each other in the correct relation as regards
their intervals.

Besides the pitch of the note there is another
factor on which the correct recognition of sounds
particularly depends, namely the colour of the sound.
Indeed, there are only very few of those endowed with
perfect pitch who can claim the distinction of possessing this faculty independent of sound colour ; most of
these persons can only rely on recognizing sounds of a
certain specific colour.

Owing to external circumstances, I could make but

few experiments with Erwin concerning this interesting question, but I was able to establish, beyond doubt, the fact that in Erwin's case perfection of musical ear is independent of sound colour. The division of sounds into recognizable and unrecognizable ones, which von Kries established when investigating his own abilities in this direction, does not exist in our case.[1]

I demonstrated by my experiments that Erwin recognizes sounds struck on stringed instruments both as to quality and pitch. With the same accuracy he judges sounds given by bells and glasses, whistled notes and high piping sounds, such as motor-horns and shrill signal-whistles.

Even the recognition of vocal sounds needed no appreciable time or reflection. He placed notes sung to him in varying heights by bass, tenor and soprano voices quite accurately, also notes sung or whistled by himself.

In addition, I made experiments with wind instruments. I tested him with notes played on the following instruments—clarinet, basset horn, basse-clarinet, oboe, English horn, bassoon, double-bassoon, trumpet, bugle, and trombone. The notes were taken from the entire range of the registers of the respective instruments. The correctness of the replies and the time taken to recognize the various notes were not influenced in any appreciable way by the fact that the instruments employed differed entirely from each other as regards the colour of the sounds emitted by them.

[1] Kries, J., "Über das absolute Gehör.", *Zeitschr. für Psychologie und Physiologie der Tinnesorgane*, vol. 3, p. 25 f.

It has, accordingly, been established by these experiments that Erwin is gifted *with a sense of absolute pitch quite independent of the colour of the sounds heard.*

An incident occurred which is very characteristic of Erwin's sense of pitch, and deserves to be recorded for the sake of its universal importance, as it illustrates a difficulty, well-known, but rarely appreciated, with which persons possessing this gift have occasionally to contend.

I went with Erwin to call on a family of our acquaintance. We had hardly entered the music-room before he went to the piano and struck a few chords. "The piano is tuned wrong", he exclaimed, "it is a semitone too low. It is really impossible to play on it." Nevertheless it appeared that the wrongly-tuned piano gave him great pleasure, for he struck some more chords and, in each case, stated their key. I then asked him to play something to us. He began to play a piece by Bach, written in C major. Although he was evidently irritated by the fact that, owing to the mistuning of the instrument, the piece sounded as if it was written in B major, he went on playing it. At first it went fairly well, but suddenly he halted, and, while one hand continued playing correctly, the other hand involuntarily passed on to the C sharp major keys. He immediately corrected himself and finished the piece unwillingly. He then tried to perform a prelude in G major by Bach. But in this he succeeded still worse. I suggested to him simply to transpose the prelude to A flat major, in order, at least, to hear it correctly in G major. He tried but did not succeed.

Certain pieces also, which, at other times, he could transpose into any key without a mistake and with the greatest ease, he was only able to play with great difficulty on the wrongly-tuned piano, and, even then, not without mistakes.

This occurrence does not need any explanation for a musician. I will only remark, that every key struck on the piano brings a disillusionment, for the player expects that the sound heard will be that of the note represented by the key; instead of this, he is always disappointed. If, on the other hand, he tries to transpose, he is bound to focus his attention on the expectation of a higher pitch. He strikes the keys according to these "transposed" images, expects when he plays C, to hear C sharp, and is now just as disappointed as before to hear C, instead of C sharp.

O. Abraham reports similar instances in his paper on perfect pitch.[1] A lady gifted with this faculty wished to play the first movement of the *C sharp minor Sonata* by Beethoven on a piano which was tuned much too low. She was unable to endure this "mood-picture" when played in C minor, it being inseparably connected in her mind with the key of C sharp minor. She, therefore, played it in the original key, although, in order to do so, she had to overcome great technical difficulties.

In the case of Erwin, the extent to which he was hampered by his perfect ear showed itself in an even more interesting manner when I asked him to improvise

[1] Abraham, O., "Das absolute Tonbewusstsein", *Sammelbände der internationalen Musikgesellschaft*, 1901.

something on the wrongly-tuned piano. He tried repeatedly but never succeeded. After a few unsuccessful attempts he had to give it up entirely.

A singer gifted with perfect pitch has to contend with similar difficulties when asked to sing a piece in a higher or lower key than the original one, whereas singers who do not possess this faculty, and only let themselves be guided by the intervals, experience no trouble of this kind. In the same way, it often becomes impossible for a singer with perfect pitch to perform in an unaccompanied chorus, because he is unable to follow those slight alterations of pitch which inevitably occur during the performance.

RECOGNITION OF INTERVALS

Another of the objects of my investigation was to ascertain the degree of accuracy shown by Erwin in recognizing intervals. I soon established the fact that he invariably recognized every kind of musical interval and gave each one its musical name. In order to arrive at a correct estimate of his power of judging intervals, I asked him to find on a "Sound Variator" the major second, the major third, the fourth, fifth, and the octave of a given note, the number of vibrations of which was 450. With this 450 vibration he connected, as successive major second the sound 508 (instead of $506\cdot2 =$ major whole tone, or $505\cdot1 =$ temperate whole tone), as succ. gr. third 567 (instead of $562\cdot5$), as succ. fourth 600 (perfect), as succ. fifth 677 (instead of 675) and as succ. octave 900 (perfect).

ANALYSIS OF CHORDS

I now passed on to the investigation of his power of recognizing and analysing chords, i.e. reducing them to their component parts. In the first of these experiments I tested him with triads and others composed of three notes, beginning with the common chords of the various keys, and their inversions, and also inverted chords. These experiments were carried out in order to test Erwin's capacity for recognizing chords, both with regard to their *genus* and their *key*.

Erwin, in the majority of cases, called the triads played to him correctly by their musical names, but it occasionally happened also that instead of their names he gave the names of their components. But the fact that he did this must not lead to the conclusion that he obtained his results by consciously resolving the triad. He merely sometimes called chords by their names and sometimes by the names of their components. If I asked him to call the chords by their names, he did so, this having no effect on the length of time he took to give his verdict. That he should have actually heard the individual notes separately is out of question, for the simple reason that the period occupied in forming the judgment was so short that there was not time to do more than recognize the chord and formulate the answer. Erwin, in fact, recognized the triads, *by their characteristic total impression*, and thus was able to repeat immediately the names of the individual notes of which they were composed.

The experiments described above refer only to the

register between C and a^4. The judgment passed on common chords in a lower region, between B_1 and B_2 was much less certain ; indeed he often failed to recognize the triads as such at all, thinking on the contrary, that they were complicated discords, and he often gave the names of a whole series of sounds which he thought he had heard, amongst which, however, the notes really played were also to be found. For a musician, this does not need any explanation, for experiments with low notes, without special practice in this direction, are always apt to lead to such a result, especially if the chords are not played on a particularly good instrument. It did sometimes happen, even in this region, that some of the chords were correctly recognized, for instance, the triads of E_1 flat, G_1, B_1 flat, or D_1, F_1 sharp, A_1, etc. When, in order to check this experiment, I occasionally made use of the beautiful, well-rounded tones of a Steinway piano, I obtained much better results.

In a further series of experiments I have played to Erwin some of the more usual discords of over three notes (chords of the seventh and ninth and their inversions) and I convinced myself that Erwin was capable of recognizing and naming them correctly, and also of reducing them to their component parts without difficulty. The chords were struck once, sharply, and Erwin's verdicts were given immediately without reflection and with perfect confidence. One characteristic of the boy's performance was that during these experiments he always smiled in a superior manner, the tasks put before him being so easy to him that he did not take them seriously.

Finally I wished to ascertain the limits of his capacity for analysing sound-combinations. To this end, I offered him sound-combinations of an unusual kind, thorough discords, almost amounting to mere noise. In the majority of cases the chords were simply struck sharply, in some cases they were held until Erwin had given his verdict. In the latter case, therefore, analysis took place as the result of an immediate impression. In the former it was not carried out during the duration of the sounds entirely by ear, but must have been based chiefly on primary memory, the chord, after its sound had ceased, having to be retained in the mind until the analysis was completed. It happened sometimes, however, that the verdict was given so long after the playing of the test (sometimes more than seven seconds later), that the analysis could not possibly have taken place by the aid of primary memory, but only on the basis of the reproduction of previous perceptions. Whether in these cases the elements of the sounds heard were reproduced singly, or whether the verdict was based on the total impression made by the combination of sounds, is a question which could only be answered satisfactorily as the result of a separate inquiry, but it may safely be assumed that it would be out of question for sound-combinations of so meaningless and wild a kind to leave an aggregate and individual impression.

Particular stress must be laid on the fact that whenever the sound-combinations submitted were particularly complicated, or consisted of a great number of notes, Erwin divided the tone-combination into several—usually into two parts—and tried to conceive and identify each of the parts separately. I draw this conclusion from the fact that, before uttering his judgment, he often placed the fingers of the right or the left hand in positions corresponding to the separate parts, and, when enumerating the sounds, always made a pause once in the enumeration. Otherwise the identifying of the sounds was always effected quickly, beginning with the lowest and working upwards.

In these experiments Erwin performed remarkable feats, *which have rarely been equalled.* In order to be able to compare the capacity of the child with that of certain musicians particularly noted for the acuteness of their musical ear, I, first of all, tested him with the experiments Stumpf carried out in connection with the excellent 'cellist, David Popper.

The following five difficult combinations were employed, every chord being struck only once sharply on the piano.

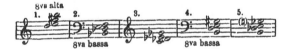

Popper did not succeed in solving the tone-combination 1 ; in the case of the chord 2, he could only give the name of the highest note ; the chords 3 and 4 were analysed correctly ; and, in the case of chord 5, the lowest note only was named.

I now played these tone-combinations to Erwin under the same experimental conditions. The notes of the chord, 1, 3, 4 and 5 were correctly given by him.   The analysis of the chord 2 was also successful, with the exception of one note, namely the deepest note B_1 flat, which he failed to identify.   But when I drew his attention to the point, I could nearly always make Erwin distinguish low notes in a chord which he had not previously noticed.

I must point out here that in the case of the multiple chord 4, Erwin was under the impression that he had heard a D sharp in addition to the notes actually struck; his statement was B, D, D sharp, E, G sharp. I should like to deal more thoroughly with this point.

For instance, it occasionally happened that Erwin, when analysing discords, gave a greater number of notes than were actually contained in the chords. These discrepancies may be divided into two groups.

1. A note is named twice, i.e. the upper octave of one note in the chord is added.   Such cases only occur when the notes of the sound complex extend over a large compass, as in the following examples :—

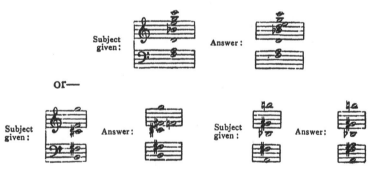

or—

This inaccuracy is probably due to the fact that Erwin hears the upper octave as the first harmonic of one of the components of the chords.

Not only octave duplications, but also octave triplications occurred sometimes.   I noticed this two or three times during my investigations.   Thus, for instance, the following combinations of four notes were played :—

The answer given was :—

In connection with these errors it was of interest to discover whether Erwin was capable of picking out by ear any octaves or double octaves actually occurring in a rapidly-played combination of notes.

Among others I played him the following multiple chords :—

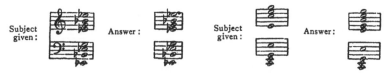

2. It was further noticeable that, in the case of the discords, he heard, besides the notes actually given, one, and sometimes—but only on rare occasions —two extra notes, which generally lay one semitone

---

¹ This note may indeed really have been present in the shape of the differential tone between *d″* and the first harmonic of a°, but it seems to me more likely that Erwin supplemented the inversion *f, a, d″*, thus making it a D minor triad.

higher or lower than one of the middle notes. This note, which he imagined he heard, occurred only when the number of notes offered was very large, and, especially, when some of them lay very close to each other. In the case of sound-complexes, such as

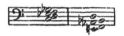

the components were stated correctly, but in the first case an E was interpolated between E flat and F, and in the second an F sharp between F and A flat. I feel certain that these inaccuracies may be attributed chiefly to insufficient concentration of attention, for, in the first place, Erwin did not repeat the mistakes when the chords were again played to him, and in the second place there were several occasions on which he resolved similar, and sometimes even identical tone-combinations without a mistake. On one occasion, for instance, the, following discords were correctly resolved :—

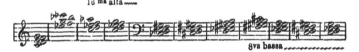

Stumpf, in his Psychology of Sound, Vol. II, p. 37, gives the following sound-groups, which are even more hideous· and dissonant, and, therefore, more difficult to resolve than those mentioned on p. 77 :—

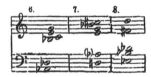

The notes of the sound - complex No. 6 were named correctly by Stumpf himself, but the lowest note was only given as probable. In the case of the chords, 7, 8, and others similar to them, he was able at any rate to state the highest note correctly.

I now submitted Erwin to the test of these tone-combinations. He analysed them correctly immediately after they had been played once to him ; only in the case of the chord 8 was the note D given twice.

In order to make the task more difficult still, and to test his musical ear with even greater severity, I transposed the chords 6 and 7 to an octave lower.

The notes were correctly given in this position also ; only in the case of the chord 6 an extra D flat was interpolated at the first trial. At the second one, two notes, B flat and D flat, were doubled. Apart from these insignificant inaccuracies, Erwin may be said to have analysed all the tone-combinations given by Stumpf correctly, so that his capacity for analysing chords by ear, compared to that of other persons who have been under observation, has proved itself to be quite extraordinary.

Owing to the kindness of Prof. von Hornbostel I was able to test Erwin's ability to analyse chords by playing to him exactly the same sound-combinations which Prof. v. Hornbostel used when investigating this capacity in the case of the young Viennese composer, E. W. Korngold, then thirteen years old.

The sound-combinations which he placed at my

F

disposal are to be found in the first line, whereas the second line contains the notes as given by Erwin at the first examination, and the third line those he gave at the second.

The components of the chords 2, 4, 5, and 9 were stated correctly at the first trial; in the case of 1 and 3 an extra note was interpolated which, however, was omitted when the test was repeated. In the case of the sound-combinations 6, 7, and 8, Erwin gave wrong notes to begin with; but, when the test was repeated, he immediately gave a correct answer.

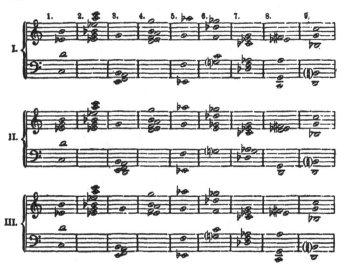

It was only later, however, that Erwin's capacity for analysis revealed itself in a most astonishing manner when, in the further course of my investigations, I played him tone-combinations which exceeded those previously given, both as regards size and disson-

ance. As an instance, Erwin analysed the following
chords :

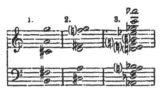

The chords 1 and 2 were analysed correctly the first
time they were played. The combination 3 was resolved
after the first short test as A flat, D flat, E, A, F flat, G,
B flat, B ; after the second long presentation as A flat,
D flat, F, B flat, G, B flat, B, A flat, E, E flat, G, C, E.
Of the thirteen notes of the chord ten were named correctly, three were doubled, and only three were omitted.

After a lapse of two years, in the year 1912, I submitted Erwin to *the same tests*. These experiments
produced still better results than those of 1910.

This may be explained, I believe, simply by the
increase in his capacity for concentration. All the
chords printed here were correctly analysed by Erwin
the first time they were played to him. The components
of the sound - complex 8 were given correctly at the
original pitch as well as when transposed an octave
higher or lower.

The examples quoted show, in fact, that Erwin's
capacity for resolving multiple chords has hardly ever,
until now, been equalled.[1]

[1] When Erwin, in 1915, spent some time in Berlin, he was examined by
Professors Stumpf and von Hornbostel. They fully confirmed my results,
and told me that Erwin's sense of absolute pitch and his capacity for analysing
chords by ear proved quite marvellous.

7. Transposing, Reading at Sight, Playing from the Score, Musical Transcription

TRANSPOSING

THE gift of perfect pitch bears close relation to the ability to transpose musical pieces into different keys, an art in which Erwin excelled as early as in his seventh year. He transposed one-part pieces, and simpler kinds of music in more parts, into any key faultlessly, and with great ease. Thus he played the *Organ Prelude in C minor* by J. S. Bach in C sharp minor and F sharp minor, in the same tempo and with just as fine an interpretation as in the original key. He transposed the *D major Sonata* by Kuhlau, *op*. 55, No. 5, into, among other keys, F sharp major B major, A flat major, E flat major and B flat major with perfect accuracy. In the same way he succeeded in transposing the two-part *Prelude No. 8*, by Bach, as well as some sonatas by Haydn. The Rondo in G major from the *G minor Sonata* by Beethoven, *op*. 49, No. 1, was also excellently transposed, *at sight*, into F sharp major and C sharp major.

It may be mentioned here that it seemed to make very little difference to Erwin when transposing a piece he knew well, and had learnt by heart, whether he had the music before him or not. If, however, there were complicated movements in the middle parts he found transposing difficult, and he was sometimes even unable to carry out the task. Thus, for instance, when I placed the *Organ Prelude in G minor* by Bach before him, asking him to transpose it into C sharp minor, he proceeded quite well until the ninth bar, where the piece suddenly becomes more complicated, the parts working against each other, and from here onwards difficulties arose which he was unable to overcome.

When I examined him again at the age of ten in April 1913, I found that his talents for transposing had developed considerably. He was now able to transpose two-part inventions, by Bach, at first sight into any desired key, and without the smallest difficulty. Thus, for instance, he transposed the *Prelude in E minor*, *No. 5*, into B flat minor, and that in *E major*, *No. 6*, into B flat major, each of them an augmented fourth higher, without mistakes and in the tempo indicated. Out of the 15 three - part Inventions by Bach, Erwin transposed quite a number into any desired key; being especially successful in the case of those which were already known to him. Among others, the Invention in D minor, No. 4, was transposed into G sharp minor and F sharp minor, and the Invention in G minor, No. 11, perhaps the most difficult and complicated of them all, into various keys, in each case excellently. These feats are worthy of consideration, owing to the fact that Erwin was not in the habit of transposing of his own accord.

READING AT SIGHT

Erwin's sight-reading was quite excellent. As early as in his seventh year this ability manifested itself in a most striking manner. Two years later, the dexterity and exactitude with which he read pieces of music previously unknown to him for the first time, in the tempo indicated, were quite wonderful, and the pieces were from the first admirably interpreted. Thus, for instance, he played the Fifth Intermezzo by Schumann, which at that time was still unknown to him, at sight without making any mistakes and in the right tempo. He also accompanied songs by Brahms admirably at sight. At the time of my last investigation in 1913 it did not embarrass him to play Beethoven and Mozart Symphonies for four hands at sight. He also played, at the first attempt, the piano parts of trios and quartets, showing an admirable power of interpretation, a fact I verified in the case of the *E flat major Quartet* by Beethoven. Professional musicians who played chamber music with him were amazed at the musical feeling, precision, and artistic understanding which he showed when reading at sight.

PLAYING FROM FULL SCORE

For some time Erwin, under the direction of Leo Weiner, had practised playing from full score, and although, in this short space of time, he had had but little training, he had already made such progress that, as an instance, he read the score of Tchaikovsky's *Fourth Symphony* quite excellently, although all the

practice he had previously had was confined to a few
symphonies by Mozart and Beethoven.   When asked
to reproduce, from the score, the parts for particular
groups of instruments only, such as, for instance, those
of the wood—wind, brass, or the string quintet, he
succeeded in doing so quite correctly and without the
slightest difficulty.   The speed with which he learned
to play from full score, his whole behaviour during the
performance and the joy and enthusiasm he evinced,
pointed clearly to his very strong feeling for instrumental music.

Writing Music

It is perhaps here that mention should be made
of the very early age at which Erwin began writing
music, and the dexterity and assurance with which he
handled this task while still in childhood.   I have
seen a piece by him (*On the Death of a Little Bird*) which
he wrote down, almost faultlessly, at the beginning of
his sixth year, at a time when he had hardly learnt to
write the letters of the alphabet.   The mistakes that
occurred were, for the most part, either orthographical
or consisted of omissions of slight importance.   Errors
as regards the time value of notes he hardly ever made
at that time.   The pieces written in his seventh and
eighth years show a thorough grasp of legato marks,
staccato marks, and pauses ; and he uses the marks of
accentuation correctly.   As time went on he began to
produce more and more complicated compositions,
and the writing of these made still greater demands
upon him, but Erwin always showed himself equal to

the task. At the age of nine he already wrote music quickly and easily, and even the most complicated construction and metre did not cause him any difficulty. With one exception, all the works published in the Appendix were written by him. I copied them directly from his manuscripts and I reproduce them exactly as I found them, so that the reader may judge for himself of the correctness of Erwin's notation.

8. Erwin's Musical Memory

I COME now to the question of Erwin's musical memory. I thought it necessary to investigate this by the aid of precise experiments, for it is of great importance with regard to artistic production. It is interesting to discover whether any relation, and, if so, what kind of relation, exists between creative imagination and intuition on one side, and activity of memory on the other. It would, however, be too far removed from my present purpose to discuss this question in detail. It will be generally admitted, however, that the various different qualities that are embodied in the gift for memorizing, such as, for instance, the diversity of types of memory, the strength of the impression received, the degree of accuracy in remembering, the illusions of memory, the power of recognizing something already familiar, the rôle played by this quality of "familiarity," etc., must undoubtedly influence creative activity, which after all is, to a certain extent, based upon the reproduction of actual experience. A reliable memory is invaluable .to a composer; with it he knows that the leading themes and motives in a musical work of some length will always be stored, ready, in his memory. A good memory will save him from involuntarily incorporating the ideas of others into his compositions.

At the time of my first experiments, made in

January 1910, I was unable thoroughly to confirm the statements made by Erwin's parents concerning his stupendous feats of memory. I did, however, establish the fact that Erwin, with the greatest ease, memorized melodious pieces harmonized in a simple manner. Pieces which his teacher asked him to learn were reproduced by him without the aid of notes after very few repetitions. Also, he had no difficulty in retaining a great number of operatic airs in his memory, and he learned them in a very short time. I noticed however, that, as a rule, only the melodies without the harmonies were reproduced without mistake. In the case of musical pieces of a strange character, such as melodies with complicated accompaniment and peculiar harmonies, his memory did not prove itself equal to the task. In order to give instances showing the limitations of his ability in such cases I will quote a few examples here.

Out of a four-part theme by Vittoria, repeated to him three times, Erwin was only able to reproduce the first four bars. The test was made acoustically.[1] The first few bars of the homophonous principal theme of the *Danse Sacrée* by Debussy were played to Erwin several times in succession. Owing to the strange character of the melody and rhythm he was unable to reproduce it, until at last I allowed him to play the theme through himself. He was also unable to reproduce the first four bars of *Weyla's Song* by Hugo Wolf,

---

[1] We speak of a test being made acoustically, when the test-material is played by the investigator, so that the person on whom the experiment is made only listens, and accordingly fixes the piece in his memory through audition merely. A visual (optic) test is that in which a piece is learnt merely by reading the notes.

played to him and repeated several times in succession. In the case of another song by H. Wolf (*Verborgenheit*) I only gave him the melody, but he was not able to reproduce it until I had played the harmonies as well. (The song should be compared.)

When six months later, in June 1910, a favourable opportunity occurred, I subjected Erwin's musical memory to another test.

Memory Experiment No. 1.

In order to examine .the *optical and acoustic memory* in co-operation, the following theme was placed before Erwin ; he played it through once himself, and, immediately afterwards, tried to reproduce it without the aid of the music.

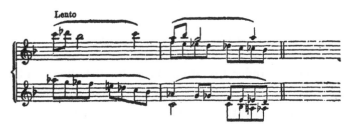

After six attempts, none of which was faultless, the experiment was broken off.[2]

[1] At this examination I put to Erwin the same questions used by Prof. von Hornbostel in his examination of E. Korngold, as to the result of which, however, I have received no information.

[2] The experiment proceeded in the following way :

After playing the piece for the first time—no reproduction was possible.
After playing it for the second time—it was wrongly reproduced.
After playing it for the third time—first bar right, second bar wrong.
After playing it for the fourth time—second bar not quite faultless yet.
A short time pause was made.
After playing it for the fifth time—wrongly reproduced.
After playing it for the sixth time—second bar wrong.

The experiment was broken off.

Memory Experiment No. 2.

In order to test Erwin's *optical memory*, he was asked to read the following theme, without playing it, until he thought he could reproduce it correctly. He then played it to me without notes.

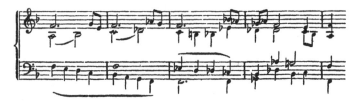

His behaviour during the memorizing of this piece was very interesting. He began by humming the melody to himself, in a subdued voice and, while doing this, he moved his fingers, as if he were playing the theme on the piano. When I noticed this, I caught hold of his right hand, but even by this means I was not able to hinder his attempts to fix the theme in his memory by motor means, attempts that continued as an accompaniment to the act of visual learning, for he went on moving, not only the fingers of the left hand that remained free, but those of his right hand also. It struck me that he was trying to imprint the treble on his memory by singing, and the lower parts by the action of playing. Sometimes, he also beat time to the tune with his feet. At each repetition he tried to memorize the theme by the aid of singing and movements of his fingers. The purpose of the experiment, which was to make him memorize by sight alone, therefore failed. The purely optical method of impressing music on the memory will, also in the case of other people, probably always turn out to be impracticable, since musical memory depends primarily on the mental assimilation of heard sounds. The theme was read by Erwin eight or nine times in succession, without a pause, and the time taken for memorizing it was six minutes and thirty seconds.[1]

Memory Experiment No. 3.

In order to investigate Erwin's *acoustic memory*, I played the following theme to him ; Erwin not being allowed to look at my fingers whilst I was playing. Immediately afterwards he was asked to play the theme without the aid of written music.[2]

Tranquillo.

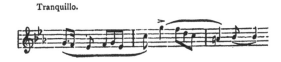

After the third attempt, the theme was reproduced without any mistake. I now made a pause of thirty seconds. After this pause I asked Erwin to repeat the theme, which he had already played once correctly. The reproduction was faultless, and even more quick and certain than on the occasion of the first faultless

[1] In this lesson, at the first attempt, the first three bars were reproduced faultlessly, and even in the fourth bar only a few mistakes in the lower parts occurred. When Erwin had read the theme twice after the first attempt he reproduced it without any mistakes.

[2] The experiment was carried out in the following way :

After the first test, reproduction was not carried out successfully, namely, there occurred a mistake in the first bar, two extra sounds were interpolated in the second, and the conclusion was also erroneous. After the second test, practically the same mistakes were made in reproduction, but after the third production, faultless reproduction was effected.

reproduction. This illustrates a well-known fact with regard to memory. It has been observed that a series of impressions are better and more firmly retained in the memory after a certain period has elapsed than directly after their assimilation. In the case of Erwin, I frequently had occasion to observe that a day or two after having learnt a certain musical piece he was able to reproduce it with greater exactitude than on the day on which he learned it. An example of this may be found on p. 95.

Memory Experiment No. 4.

This test was carried out in exactly the same manner as Experiment No. 3.

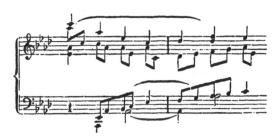

Reproduction, after the first attempt, was not fault-less. The treble was reproduced correctly, but the lower parts were wrong, additions being made by Erwin, without, however, altering the character of the theme. The experiment was repeated, but without success, and the difficulties appeared to me so great that I considered it best to break off the experiment in order not to put too great a strain on the attention and strength of the child.

Then followed a pause of five minutes. After

this opportunity of rest, I repeated the first three tests.[1]

The experiments proved that, after the pause, Erwin was able to reproduce the themes 2 and 3, which he had thoroughly assimilated, without a mistake. With regard to theme 1, he was unable to reproduce it, though I played it to him again on the piano four times in succession. Thus, even ten repetitions of this theme, the repetitions being spread over a length of time—a circumstance which is well-known to increase the effectiveness of associations—did not lead to faultless reproduction.

On the afternoon of the same day I investigated the strength of the associations formed during the morning. On Erwin's declaring that he had forgotten all the themes, I first of all asked him to play the first one, reading it from the music, twice in succession; he was able to play it immediately afterwards without the notes. Another trial with the same theme, a little later, was also perfectly successful, which confirms what I have already said on p. 94 concerning this feature of memorizing. During the morning it was impossible to get him to reproduce the theme correctly, in spite of frequent repetitions; in the afternoon, on the other hand, it was very quickly impressed upon Erwin's memory. This speed in memorizing cannot be placed entirely to the credit of the last two repetitions, but is

[1] I here wish to observe that in the experiments recorded above, the object of the investigation was immediate memory, i.e. the capacity for reproducing impressions immediately or a short time after their perception. In the experiments which follow, on the other hand, retention, or memory proper, is under examination.

greatly due to the deferred effect of the associations formed during the morning.

As to the second theme, Erwin looked at it very attentively for about twenty-eight seconds, and then reproduced it without a mistake. In the case of the third theme, he treated it in exactly the same way.

Next morning I asked Erwin to write out the three themes. He was quite ready to do so, without having to memorize them again, and wrote them down as follows :

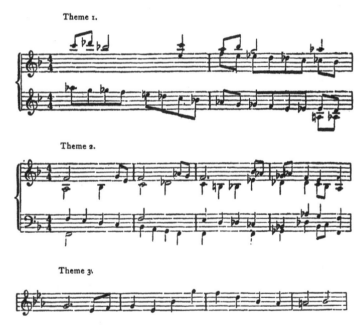

Theme 1.

Theme 2.

Theme 3.

The first theme is transcribed without a mistake, with the exception of the small deviation in the second bar of the left hand. The second is faultless, whereas the third one, which was only heard by him, was incorrectly transcribed, although it was only a one-part theme.

These results show that Erwin reproduces music very faithfully and reliably when he is not compelled to rely on his ear alone in memorizing it.

Two years after these experiments, on the 22nd of May, 1912, I tested Erwin's musical memory again, in order to ascertain how far it had developed during this time. In order to find out, first of all, whether any traces still remained of the associations established during the former tests, I made him learn the same themes with which I had tried him two years before. Although he had never repeated any of these themes (even mentally, so he declared) he was able to reproduce them correctly after repeating them once. In the case of theme 2 he did not make use even of this single repetition. It is evident, therefore, that Erwin's power of retaining in his memory themes once learnt is very remarkable.

In order to ascertain his capacity for memorizing new themes I made the following experiments :

Memory Experiment No. 5

The theme was originally selected in order to test *optical memory*. As, however, I could see from Erwin's attitude, directly after the first reading of the theme, that he would certainly not be able to commit it to memory by mere reading, I allowed him to play it through once while the visual impression was being made on his mind. The method of impression used, therefore, was, on the whole, an optical one.

G

After having read the theme through several times, Erwin played it once, then he read it again, and memorized it once more — probably in a combined auditory-motor way — and it was only then that he reproduced the first five bars, without any mistake.

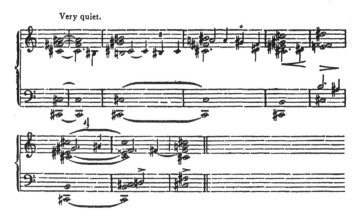

The result, therefore, was considerably better than it had been in the case of theme 1 or 2, in 1910. The present theme was three times as long as the other, and the difficulties of each may be considered practically equal. But while, in the 1910 experiment, the theme was not reproduced faultlessly after ten repetitions, on the present occasion, three repetitions were sufficient to ensure a perfect reproduction of the greater part of the theme.

Memory Experiment No. 6

Theme taken from the *Seven Seals* by Richard Strauss (*opus* 46, No. 3). Method of examination the same as in the case of Experiment No. 3. The subject of the examination was, therefore, *acoustic memory*.

At the first trial he was still very uncertain in his reproduction of the fourth and fifth bars, after the

Bright.

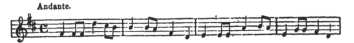

second repetition, however, the whole theme was given without a mistake. The time taken for learning it was twenty-two seconds. The result, therefore, is better in any case than that of theme 3 of the year 1910.

Memory Experiment No. 7

Scandinavian popular tune. Method of examination similar to that used in Experiment No. 2; the subject being, therefore, *visual memory*—as far as this is at all possible.

Andante.

The melody was read four times and then faultlessly reproduced. The time taken to learn it was fifty-eight seconds.

Memory Experiment No. 8

From *Electra* by Richard Strauss. Method similar to that used in the preceding experiment.

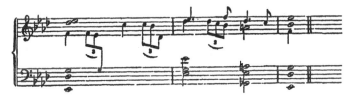

The time taken for memorizing amounted to forty seconds. At the second attempt after the theme had been put before him, it was reproduced without a mistake. Immediately afterwards he played it once again, with extraordinary speed.

Six days later, on the 28th of May, 1912, I repeated these experiments with Erwin, in order to test his powers of retention. Theme 5, after a single repetition, went as well as on the occasion of the last experiment, namely without a mistake except in the last four bars; the others (6, 7, and 8) he played faultlessly without any preceding repetition. These results prove that Erwin's musical memory had developed in a remarkable manner during the last two years, as, two years before, a pause of from four to five hours would have been quite sufficient to make reproduction without a repeated hearing impossible.

A year after the experiments referred to, on the 20th of April, 1913, I tested Erwin's musical memory once more. First of all, I ascertained that he was able to play the greater part of the themes I had asked him to learn three years before and in the preceding year, without my having to repeat them. At my request, he played the greater part of the themes in quick succession and, as regards the others, which he did not remember immediately, he only required to read them through once in order to be able to reproduce them.

The following are further experiments which I carried out with Erwin in order to ascertain his capacity for learning musical pieces and the power of his memory.

Memory Experiment

Theme on p. 94.   As in the case of *Memory Experiment No.* 3, the acoustic memory was again tested.   I had already used this theme with Erwin in 1910, but at that time could get no result.   He also attempted it on another occasion, but without success.   This time he succeeded in reproducing it correctly after six repetitions.

Further, I repeated the *Memory Experiment No.* 5 in which Erwin, the year before, had only been able to memorize part of the theme, and in which it had been necessary to aid the visual method of learning by the acoustic-motoric method.   It appeared that Erwin had in course of time practically forgotten the first five bars which he had learnt the year before, as it took a comparatively long time to impress the fourth and fifth bars upon his mind.   The method used was the visual one, as in the case of *Experiment No.* 2.   I was not able to ascertain how many times Erwin had read the theme, for he divided it into small parts, learning each fraction separately, and then associating it with the adjoining ones.   All I could establish definitely was the time taken to memorize the theme.   In the beginning the theme was read over for a period of three minutes, forty seconds.   This did not result in a complete reproduction of the whole theme, only the first five bars being reproduced without mistake.   Another two minutes, twenty seconds devoted to memorizing resulted in an almost faultless reproduction of the whole theme.   Finally it was read over for a period of thirty seconds, the result being a perfectly faultless reproduction. The total time taken to memorize the theme amounting, therefore, to six minutes, thirty seconds.

Erwin's extraordinary power of retaining musical themes in his memory was manifested in a particularly striking manner two weeks later, when he proved himself able to reproduce both themes faultlessly, without any repetition.

Since the child had already shown such an excellent memory for extraordinary sequences of sounds and harmonies, it was only to be expected that he would be even more successful in memorizing musical pieces, which were not only more fluent in character, but also in more immediate connection with his preceding musical experiences. They were, therefore, familiar to him in form and substance and were easily assimilated as part of a cycle of corresponding impressions.

In the year 1910, I had tested Erwin already with a number of easy and melodious musical pieces, asking him to learn them, and achieving excellent results. On one occasion he mastered the *G major Waltz* by Chopin (*Valse* 7), which he had not previously known, after five repetitions. In 1912 I gave him the first twenty-eight bars of Schumann's "Intermezzo," *opus* 4, No. 5. I asked him to play it through first, then try to perform it again without looking at the notes and, in case he found himself unable to continue, I told him to avail himself of the music which lay before him. In the first attempt this help was needed twelve times, and in the second, only five. When he had

played through the piece once more it went perfectly
correctly. After a lapse of six days he was still able
to reproduce the "Intermezzo" correctly, with the exception of a few mistakes in the accompaniment. He
studied the great "Piano Concerto" by Schumann,
opus 54, but not with the express purpose of learning it by heart, for a week and a half, playing it
not more than once a day. On one occasion, during
a lesson, it happened that his teacher had lent his
copy to some one, whereupon *Erwin offered to play
his part by heart, and succeeded perfectly by doing so.*
He memorized many sonatas by Beethoven and fugues
by Bach after having repeated them three or four
times.

It is only possible to verify the amazing scope of
Erwin's memory by comparing it with that of other
musicians with the aid of comparative experiments.

With this end in view, I put the same tests to
which I had submitted Erwin to Miss Elise Láng, a
certificated piano teacher, and an excellent pianist, who
is distinguished for her sense of absolute pitch, and
her very good musical memory.

Theme 1, which Erwin was not able to reproduce
on the first day of our experiments, even after six
repetitions, was faultlessly memorized by the teacher,
after she had played it through five times.[1]

At a subsequent examination, about half an hour

[1] The experiment was carried out in the following manner : After having
played the theme through once, the pianist thought she could reproduce it,
but did not succeed in doing so. When she had performed it another time,
she reproduced bar 1 and the first two quavers of bar 2 correctly. After the
next performance, no progress was visible. After the third performance,
faultless reproduction was attained.

later, she reproduced the theme without a mistake, after having it played through once previously.

As to theme 2, which Erwin had memorized in six minutes, thirty seconds, and had then reproduced almost faultlessly, reproducing it without any mistakes after he had played it through twice, the lady pianist was able to impress it upon her mind in six sections, taking six minutes, 4 seconds, to memorize it.[1] Although the time taken by Erwin for learning the theme was a little longer, yet his feat of memory must be considered a greater one than that of the lady pianist, since he had memorized the theme in two attempts. The superiority of Erwin, however, shows itself in the fact that half an hour later he was able to reproduce the theme without a repetition, whereas the teacher had to read it through once more in order to do this.

As to theme 3, the lady pianist impressed it upon her memory after four, Erwin after three, repetitions. Half an hour later, in order to attain a faultless reproduction, another repetition was needed in the case of Miss Láng and no further repetition on the part of Erwin.

As regards theme 4, the lady pianist did not succeed in reproducing it at all after two repetitions. With

[1] The experiment was carried out as follows : After taking a time of two minutes, eighteen seconds to learn the theme, the first two bars were reproduced correctly, the others not. After a further time of two minutes, one second, the reproduction of the third bar was still incorrect, after another ten seconds, the first three bars were reproduced faultlessly, after ten seconds more, the whole theme was reproduced almost without a mistake, after thirteen seconds more there were still some difficulties about the fourth bar, and finally after another twelve seconds the theme was reproduced twice in succession without a fault.

Erwin, the results attained were slightly better (compare p. 101).

Further, as in the case of Erwin, I tested the capacity of the lady pianist for retaining the themes she learned in her memory. This examination, carried out twenty-four hours after the theme had been impressed on her memory showed the following results: Theme 1 was reproduced after one repetition, theme 2, after a period of eighteen seconds for memorizing, and theme 3 without any repetition. With Erwin, the result was a little better; it must be remembered, however, that in his case there had been a preceding examination only five hours after memorizing.

When, after a further twenty-four hours had elapsed, I repeated the experiments with the teacher, it appeared that the reproduction of themes 1 and 2 without a repetition was still impossible; and, when examined again, after a lapse of a further twenty-four hours, she was still unable to reproduce the theme without at least a cursory previous repetition of it. Erwin, on the other hand, had memorized themes 1 and 2 at the first experiment so precisely that he was able to write them out after twenty-four hours without any further repetition, and has not forgotten them to this day.

Thus, these comparative experiments have shown that Erwin's immediate musical memory, in 1910, was practically equal to that of a grown-up musician possessed of a good ear; his power of retention on the other hand,—and it is this which counts particularly in musical practice,—was at that time already much better than that of a good musician.

It has already been pointed out that Erwin's memory had greatly developed during the last few years. The progress that had been made in consequence of this development may again be best shown by comparative experiments with the lady pianist carried out with the themes 5, 6, 7, and 8.

I first asked her to read through theme No. 5, a task which occupied twenty-five seconds, and then I made her play it through once—just as Erwin had done. This had been sufficient, in Erwin's case, to make the immediate reproduction of the first five bars possible. In that of the lady pianist, however, it was necessary for her to repeat the theme on the piano six times before she was able to reproduce the first five bars without a mistake.

As to theme 6, Miss Láng memorized it in two sections, taking thirty seconds. Erwin learned it rather more quickly, in twenty-two seconds. Theme 7 had been learnt by Erwin in four sections, the whole time taken being fifty-eight seconds; the lady memorized it in four sections and in one minute, eighteen seconds. Theme 6, which Erwin had been able to impress upon his memory in two sections, taking forty seconds in which to learn it, was reproduced by Miss Láng only after six repetitions, taking three minutes, fifty-one seconds in which to memorize it.

Even then Miss Láng could not play the theme in a quick tempo, or without a certain difficulty. In order to attain the same tempo which Erwin had achieved after forty seconds, another production of the theme was necessary in her case, lasting seven seconds, including six repetitions on the piano, the reading of it from the music, and another four or five repetitions by heart.[1]

The extent to which Erwin's powers of retention had developed during these two years is shown by the comparative experiments which I carried out with Miss Láng six days after the foregoing tests. These experiments showed that theme 4 was only reproduced by the teacher after two repetitions, theme 6 after fourteen seconds in two sections, theme 7 in like manner, and theme 8 after 21·2 seconds. As has been said before, Erwin repeated the same themes faultlessly, after a lapse of six days, practically without the necessity for any further repetition.

[1] The experiment was carried out in the following manner:

After a period of memorizing of one minute, fifty-one seconds, bar 1 went faultlessly, bar 2 not quite so well.

After a further forty-seven seconds, it was still the same.

After a further fifteen seconds, bar 2 a little better.

After a further twenty-five seconds, without mistakes but uncertainly and with difficulty.

_ After a further fifteen seconds, still one mistake in bar 2, and still uncertain.

After a further eighteen seconds, without mistakes, slowly.

After a further seven seconds, without mistakes and a little more quickly.

9. Erwin as a Pianist

ERWIN'S remarkable talent as a pianist showed itself in a most striking manner at the very beginning of his regular musical education, but it did not develop evenly. From his seventh to his ninth year, his technical powers progressed steadily, but not equally. The reason for this was that, at times, the child lost interest in piano playing, and concentrated on composition. As a rule, he regarded playing the piano simply as a means to express his compositions, and he was far from experiencing any pleasure in mere virtuosity.

In his ninth year his attitude changed, owing to the fact that he began to receive systematic instruction in piano playing. He began to practise diligently and with pleasure, and applied himself earnestly to the working out of a repertoire of his own. In his eighth and ninth year he did not impress his hearers so much by his technique as by his extraordinary musical sense. Hearing him, one realized that the pieces were not merely studied and that his performance was not an imitation, modelled upon the playing of others. His rendering of the easier sonatas by Mozart and Beethoven, the inventions by Bach, Schumann, and Chopin's works for the piano, was remarkable, and the astounding degree of musical intelligence with which he conceived and performed these deeply significant compositions was very striking.

His playing was soft, tender, and flexible, when these qualities were called for by the exigencies of interpretation, and hard, sure, and passionate whenever strong accents were needed. He was never uncertain as to when melodies ought to be expressed in a singing, sustained manner, or when they should be clearly articulated. In contrapuntal themes, he used every means in his power to bring out each separate part clearly, and he never wavered for a single moment in deciding between the chief and the subordinate *motifs*.

But capable as he showed himself in his interpretation of the works of others, his great talent as an interpretative artist was only seen fully when he played his own compositions. His way of touching the keys was then different, his movements betrayed passion, his attention became absolutely concentrated on the interpretation of the piece, and even his physical strength seemed to double itself on these occasions. The powerful impression made by the child on his audience is difficult to convey, it must be seen to be realized to its full extent.

Since 1911, Erwin's capacity as a pianist advanced enormously. His playing has entirely lost any childlike character it might have possessed, his performance greatly improved as regards the variety of means at his disposal, and the brilliance and fullness of his artistic power. What is most charming in his performance is the natural way in which he plays, his strong musical sense and the modesty shown in his interpretation, in which he entirely subordinates himself to the work and the composer.   The lightness with which his fingers glide over the keys, the freshness and grace of his touch are worthy of the greatest admiration.   Technical difficulties hardly exist for him any more.   He is imbued with the truth of Schumann's words : " That which the fingers create, is a technical construction ; but that which has been sounding in the soul speaks to all and outlives the mortal body."

His inherently genuine musical nature manifests itself in his interpretation of the creations of the great masters.   His teacher may instruct him as to certain points, but it is always he, himself, who recognizes the character and meaning of the piece.   It is this indispensable gift which qualifies him to criticize piano playing.   It is really wonderful to observe in how reasoned a manner and with how precise a vision he discusses the qualities and defects of concert players. If he pronounces any judgment, contrary to that of other people, he does not cling to his opinion in the headstrong, self-willed manner of a child, but states the reasons which prompted him to form it.

It was very interesting to hear Erwin's criticisms at a concert given by D'Albert.   He said that D'Albert had interpreted the *Appassionata* so excellently that there was no room for criticism, but, on the other hand, he was so dissatisfied with the way Schumann's *Carneval* had been performed, that he left the concert.   In fact, D'Albert played the *Carneval* at such a furious pace that the various parts of the suite became almost unintelligible.   Its picturesque and melodious character

was altogether blurred, its grace and delicacy vanished,
only the strength and power of the style were brought
out in a masterly manner. Erwin's opinion was that
D'Albert was acting on an entirely erroneous theory,
being under the impression that the suite was simply
illustrative of a mad and merry carnival. On the
contrary, there are numbers in it which have nothing
whatever to do with a carnival feast, they are soft and
melodious, often earnest and sad, then again mad and
joyful. No two of the numbers contained in this work
should be played alike, each one of them contains
a different degree of feeling. This view of Erwin's
coincides in a remarkable manner with that of the
composer himself, which, later on, I happened to find
in his own works. Schumann, in fact, writes as follows
about the origin of his *Carneval*, on the occasion of its
performance by Liszt for the first time, at Leipzig : " I
will only say a few words about this composition,
which owes its birth to chance. The name of a little
town (Asch) where a musical friend of mine lived, was
composed wholly of letters which represent notes on the
musical scale, and which happened also to be contained
in my own name ; thus originated one of those musical
puns which have been known to us since the days of
Bach. One piece after the other was produced, just at
the moment when the Carnival of 1835 was in full
swing and, moreover, in an earnest mood, and under
peculiar conditions. I later gave the pieces titles and
christened the whole collection *Carneval*".[1] This quota-
tion needs no further comment ; it is particularly charac-

[1] Rob. Schumann, *Gesammelte Schriften*, vol. II, p. 240.

teristic of Erwin's power of judgment that he did not allow himself to be influenced by the titles, with their reminiscences of Carnival, such as Pierrot, Arlequin, Colombine, etc.

As a child, one of Erwin's greatest successes as a pianist was his interpretation of the *Concerto in E flat major* by Beethoven. The audience was transfixed at the masterly lucidity of the boy's playing; they were astonished at his extraordinary finish, the fullness of his tone and the genuine beauty of his interpretation. He achieved great success at private concerts in Budapest and in Vienna, as well as at one he gave before the King and Queen of England, and English society in London. In London he made the acquaintance of Arthur Nikisch, who could not find words to praise the musical achievements of the boy sufficiently highly. Other musical celebrities also, who heard him in Berlin at that time, expressed their admiration of the little fellow to me. I, of course, attach special importance to the opinions of these men, because they proved that my own judgments were not too personal or dictated by excess of good-will. In any case, careful study of the documents, data, proofs, etc. contained in this book will convince the reader of the impartiality of my judgment.

What Erwin has already accomplished as a pianist justifies us in the assumption that he will never be counted among the "infant prodigies", in the current meaning of the word. In these "infant prodigies" there is generally a lack of equilibrium between the technical gifts and the musical sense, and whatever success they may achieve in the interpretation of musical works is due to imitation and is not derived from an inner, personal source, but from outside inspiration. These virtuosos generally lose their power and vanish, a fact which is all the more strange, as external circumstances are usually favourable to their musical development.

For this reason, the impression they produce is generally only a fleeting one, since it is due more to our interest in abnormal things rather than to real musical enjoyment. We are only too prone to endow the musical feats of a prodigy of this kind with a higher artistic value than he deserves, for the stupendous technique and personal charm of the child may have an enormous suggestive effect.

Children who possess a real gift of music stand far above these "infant prodigies." I am fully convinced that Erwin will never belong to this class of virtuosos for, even at the time of my investigations, his interpretation did not lack the creative quality, which is a distinctive feature of genuine reproductive artists.

H

10. Improvizing and Modulating

ERWIN'S creative activity may be divided into two parts; improvizing and composing in the strict sense of the word. During the first period of his musical development, between his fifth and seventh year, Erwin improvized more than he composed. If a theme occurred to him, he at once went to the piano, and began to improvize on it. At this time he did not even know the first rules of the theory of composition, and had heard and learnt but little, and, therefore, could hardly base his improvizations consciously on any fixed musical form, but his performances were rich in significant and unsignificant, trivial and witty musical ideas. He was at the same time genuine and ungenuine, original and imitative.

Yet, some of these improvizations showed greater uniformity, and were nobler in style, than the spontaneous productions of most beginners.

When Erwin sat down to improvize he often produced striking musical forms which, even at that time, pointed to the existence of deeply-rooted musical emotions. On these occasions one had the impression that a wonderful world of emotions was seeking for expression in these groping, searching attempts.

It is a remarkable fact that the improvizations of this period, although they did not reach the level of the written compositions as to form, accomplishment, and harmonization, on the other hand, greatly surpassed the latter as regards imagination, colour and sonority. This is partly explained by the fact that, at that time, Erwin had not sufficient perseverance and patience to write down his music, so that, when transcribing, he confined himself to that which was most important and easiest to put on paper.   Therefore, the ability for composition he possessed at that time and the wealth of his imagination may be more justly gauged by his improvizations than by his compositions.   At that time I often heard him improvize or extemporize freely on the piano, and, I must say, I was less struck by the creations themselves than by the manner in which he produced them.   When he sat in this way before the piano, thoughtful and perfectly engrossed by the music, I had the impression that I was in the presence, not of a child, but of an artist of deep insight.

Erwin usually succeeded better with improvizations on his own themes than on those of others.   Occasionally, however, he achieved admirable success with the latter.   For instance, when he was just six years old, we gave him a simple pastoral theme, and asked him to improvize, first of all, a funeral march on it.   He executed this task excellently.   The funeral march was composed of several sections.   The first began with the original theme slightly modified to suit a funeral march, and while powerful harmonies thundered deep in the bass, the theme slowly mounted upwards.   Then followed a repetition of the theme, this time in the lyrical manner, on the sub-dominant. Towards the end heavy, measured chords mounted steadily and slowly, and, like clear - sounding arpeggios on the harp, accompanied the theme, which died away in the depths.

Afterwards, Erwin was asked to improvize a children's song on the same theme. This was the most astounding feat he performed, at that time, in my hearing.

Without reflecting, he at once started an allegro. The melody was heard, fresh and joyful in treatment. The piece increased in strength and tempo, and pretty little figures ran up and down the scale. It was a merry, joyful medley of sound, full of life and freshness. The theme was never lost ; once it was brought out on the sub-dominant, then suddenly dropped again whilst the right hand performed mad gambols in octaves.

I am sorry that it was impossible to make a record of these improvizations. As a specimen piece from this period I print on p. 140 a theme which Erwin, after having heard it for the first time, developed in the manner given there.

In the period of development that followed Erwin did not improvize to any such extent as in former times, and, at the end of this period, his improvizations were not in any way superior to his compositions. They were no reliable guide to his creative capacity, and only bore witness to his spontaneity, his quick-wittedness, and the wealth of his imagination. It appeared also that improvizations which required a

stronger concentration of attention and greater amount
of discipline suited his nature better, at that stage of his
development, than mere extemporization which gave
his imagination full swing.

But these more serious improvizations vanished as
soon as they were born; for it rarely happens that an
improvization is repeated and worked out, and, still
more rarely, is it transcribed.

In order to give an idea of Erwin's capacity for
improvization, I print on p. 141 and p. 142 two on the
same theme, executed at different times.

Erwin's attitude, when composing, was quite
different. He then set to work with a fixed purpose
and often with a preconceived plan. The thoughts
generally occurred to him during a walk, or were the
result of deliberate reflection, more rarely they came
when extemporizing. The development and execution
of his thoughts generally took place at the writing-
table, less frequently on the piano. The pieces which
he occasionally composed when sitting at the piano
were only of the character of sketches, and cursory and
provisional in type. Only when they were written
down did they attain their final form. The fact must
also be emphasized that the motor element found its
expression in gestures of playing, when composing at
the writing-desk, as well as on the occasion of the
actual transcription of the composition. The importance of these playing gestures in composition should
be thoroughly investigated. It would, for instance, be
interesting to ascertain the rôle played by these gestures
when they are used as an accompaniment to musical

imagination and made to take the place of similar movements on the piano.   Perhaps, among others, we might establish the fact that they aid the creative activity of the imagination (in the same way in which the action of piano playing stimulates the productive faculties), and further, that, subconsciously, they may largely increase the power to reproduce a series of acoustic impressions, or it may be that they help the composer to strengthen the clearness, distinctness, and vividness of half-faded acoustic impressions, etc.

The art of modulation is of the greatest importance in connection with improvization.   I studied Erwin's talent for modulation in his compositions, and I also made it the subject of a separate inquiry.

He began to modulate as early as in his sixth year. Of course, at that time, these modulations were only made between keys which stood in close relationship to each other.   Thus, for instance, in a charming piece for the piano, composed in 1909, Erwin modulated from one minor key to the minor key of the sub-dominant; in another case, from a major key to both dominants. In another piece, composed in the same year, we find a modulation from one minor key to the major key of the dominant, but the transition is not satisfactory.   In the compositions he produced in his eighth and ninth year the modulations were partly carried out in an ordinary way, and partly with great freedom and in a very irregular manner.   Erwin made use of deceptive cadences very early, and, even at the beginning of his productive career, he was able occasionally to utilize complex harmonies for the purpose of modulation.

I then tried to draw his attention to the significance and beauty of modulation, and to this end I played him, first of all, sound-groups with various modifications, then deceptive cadences and progressions, etc., asking him to reproduce them by heart after having heard them once. These experiments proved that modulations did not yet occupy his attention, though he himself used them at times, for, in the case of these themes, only the melody was grasped correctly and without mistakes, whereas the modulations were badly reproduced.

Therefore, as this method did not prove the right one, I tried another.

I gave him a theme in C major, and asked him to develop it, and conclude it in G sharp minor. He varied the theme for a time, suddenly modulated from C major to G minor and then by an enharmonic inversion of a chord passed abruptly to G sharp minor. In another experiment he was asked to modulate from a theme in E flat major to D major. He went on extemporizing for a long time in E flat major and finally modulated chromatically into D major.

These experiments were carried out when Erwin was six years old. Since then he has modulated freely in his compositions as well as in his improvizations, his mode of procedure being apparent in the examples I have published.

The slow progress he made in the art of modulation may be due to the fact that in the first stages of his musical education he received no training in the theory of harmony or counterpoint, although he was continually asking for it. No other course remained open to him, consequently, but to concentrate on the great masters, and to try to wrest from them the secrets of composing. It was not until the spring of 1912 that he received regular instruction in the theory of harmony. Since that time Erwin made great progress in the construction of musical phrases and in harmonizing. From this time onwards mistakes in part-writing and harmonizing occurred less frequently. He paid such close attention to the movements of the individual parts that consecutive octaves, and open or hidden consecutive fifths, etc., if they occurred, were the result of an oversight. He also avoided other violations of the classical theory of harmony, but when it seemed to him that an effect could be produced only by the sacrifice of traditional theory, he did not hesitate for a moment to deviate from the rule. But he always gave conclusive reasons for each deviation. It should here be remarked, however, that his part-writing was at that time still far from perfect. If, in fact, we had wished then to compare his capacity in this respect with that of adult pupils, we should have had to class him with those of a mediocre capacity.

I publish here, as examples, a few uncorrected modulations, which he executed on the piano, not long ago, at my request, taking practically no time for reflection. The last modulation from D flat major to E minor, which he wrote three weeks later than the others, is characteristic of his quick development and remarkable capacity for learning.

(Oct. 1913). Modulation from C major to D flat major.

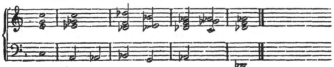

From C sharp minor to A flat major.

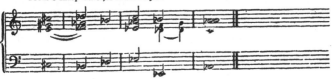

From C major to B major.

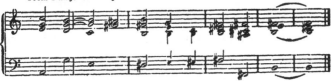

(Nov. 1913). From D flat major to E minor.

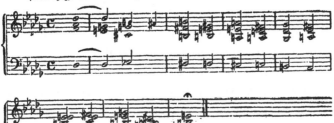

The systematic instruction which Erwin received at that time was assimilated with the utmost ease. He acquired the necessary knowledge quickly and without difficulty. As his teachers reported, it was generally sufficient to show or explain anything to him once, after which he not only understood it, but grasped it in such a manner that, when the occasion arose, he was able to utilize it. This was strikingly apparent in his improvizations. It is, however, possible that he was at that time incapable of acquiring certain necessary branches of knowledge, which were too far in advance of his existing musical development and the acquisition and use of which demanded a riper and more mature mentality than he then possessed.

As an instance, after a few attempts his harmony master had to give up his plan of teaching counterpoint to him in a *systematic manner*, for he recognized that Erwin, in spite of his great musical intelligence, was still unable to grasp the more abstruse principles of counterpoint, such as the laws governing countermovements. To impress those principles in a mechanical way on his mind was, of course, out of question. He also appeared to be unable to grasp the instruction given to him concerning the fingering on the violin, in spite of a thorough explanation given to him which, however, only covered general principles. He was also unable to understand, theoretically, the different principles of transposition and clef reading. These shortcomings must be ascribed partly to his youth, and partly to the difficulty he found in concentrating his attention on these subjects.

At my first investigation I had already been struck by Erwin's capacity for quick mental acquisition. The boy grasped musical ideas, signs, in fact, everything that stood in any relation to music, with astounding rapidity. He asked me once to supply him with information concerning certain instruments. On this occasion I explained the various clefs to him and gave him information on the compass of the more important instruments and the notation of the transposing instruments. When I saw him again, two days later, he spontaneously repeated everything to me that I had told him. To my great surprise, he read the notes of the transposing instruments correctly, stated with ease the sound of the written note on the transposing instrument and, conversely, indicated how it should be written for the instrument.

It might be argued that the success of this mental effort was due to the intensity of his interest and the concentration of attention which resulted from it. Those factors may certainly have been influential, but this would not in any way account for the ease and accuracy with which the child's mind assimilated musical matter. It is evident that the excellence of this intellectual performance was but a manifestation of one particular aspect of his genius. It is beyond doubt that talent has an influence on the selection of the subjects learnt, the manner of learning, the formation of associations and the quickness of perceptions, etc. As a matter of fact, Erwin's assimilation of all musical ideas was more rapid than it would have been in the case of a man less gifted as regards music.

Owing to his great talent, past and newly-acquired, musical experiences were united in an easier and more solid manner, owing to his grasp of the significance of their relations to each other. Even the most simple musical forms meant something to him, for they stimulated his imagination and engrossed his mind. The elements of musical compositions were more sharply divided from each other in his case, and yet, for this very reason, they were more speedily adapted to new combinations.

11. Compositions

WE now come to Erwin's compositions. I have left the consideration of this most conclusive evidence of his musical talent to the end for this reason : that the various factors that influenced his development as a musician, the circumstances under which it took place, the progress of his musical education, and his extraordinary mental abilities must be taken into consideration, if we are to judge his creative work fairly.

To arrive at a correct estimate of Erwin's ability as a composer would be an easy matter if it were possible to measure his works by the standards set by great masters, and gauge the value of his compositions unreservedly by simply comparing them with the works of adult composers. But this is not possible. In judging the creations of children, circumstances must be considered which, in the case of mature artists, need never be taken into account at all. Suppose, for instance, that a child, perhaps unconsciously, draws inspiration from a known source, we must assume an entirely different attitude towards it than we should towards a grown-up person who, it is fair to suppose, has an exact knowledge of existing musical literature, and in the case of whom one would certainly condemn reminiscences, and, worse, plagiarisms, even though these may be involuntary. Then again, if the young author offends against the first principles of convention and violates the laws of harmony we cannot judge him until we have ascertained whether he has ever received any instruction in the theory of composition. For mistakes which are due to the lack of a certain kind of knowledge bear no relation to the talent of a child. It is only when gross offences against the elementary laws of part-writing and harmony are committed that we are justified in doubting the musical talent of the offender. It is, therefore, necessary to proceed very cautiously when appraising the works of a child, and not to judge a young composer too severely if he is not yet familiar with all the rules. Of course, on the other hand, we must not base our estimation of a real artist on his most mediocre achievements. We must take into account his richness of thought, invention, creative impulse, and passion for work, and overlook faulty and inaccurate details, for, after all, pure harmonies, pellucid style, correct musical structure and complete mastery of counterpoint are things which may be acquired by dint of careful application and industry ; while musical inspiration, power of invention, artistic taste and poetical fervour are the birthright of talent, and cannot be learnt.

I found it impossible, at the time, to make a general critical survey of Erwin's musical compositions, for nearly all of them, with the exception of the last, were only trials, the first flights of his genius. He was still under the influence of certain great masterpieces, and, therefore, often produced work which was not entirely original. Perhaps he had not yet discovered the medium which would express his ideas in the most perfect way. He was still at the beginning of his real musical development, or, at best, in the middle of it; and would only attain the fullness of his development after the completion of his musical education, and when his first great struggles and exaltations began. Before this time arrives, the course of his musical development may change, and, though the direction of his future artistic bent seems already assured, we may still prophesy wrongly, however clear the indications may be, for it is rarely possible to predict the ultimate development of a young artist. Still, we may draw many important and interesting conclusions from the study of Erwin's works and gain a truthful impression of the greatness of his talent and the progress of his development during his youth.

Early creative work must always be considered and judged in its entirety. One must not be influenced by the fact that certain passages are unsatisfactory, and some of the transitions clumsy. This holds good, especially in the case of the longer pieces, in which there is a greater demand for broadly-developed construction, and in which the lack of adequate technical craftsmanship will be all the more felt, and this, to a much greater extent than if the work were that of a finished artist who, as a rule, can always fall back upon skill when the inspiration from which he draws his themes fails him.

The chief thing to be considered in such works is style, invention, and, when one compares several works by the same composer, the measure of progress achieved. Indeed, it may quite well happen that certain compositions which are unimpeachable from the point of view of mere technique may be essentially vulgar or trivial in style, while other works, which may be genuine artistic achievements, lack form, in spite of the fact that they belong to an incomparably more noble type of creative work.

It was characteristic of Erwin, in this respect, that his creative work should be based on that of the masters of the classical period of German music. This point must be emphasized because, unlike Erwin, the greater number of young composers follow in the steps of their most famous contemporaries, taking both their ideas and their forms of expression from them. In contrast to these, Erwin's compositions long remained almost entirely free from the influence of well-known contemporary composers, although he knew their work well and, indeed, had a high opinion of several of them. The classical composers, on the other hand, stand in intimate relation to him, a relation which is based on a natural affinity of artistic thought and expression, and it is for this reason that the older masters had such vital effect on him, and were destined to become his teachers. But this influence never degenerated into plagiarism.[1] His compositions are the expression of a free and independent imagination ; they spring from his most intimate inner conscious-

[1] Yet sometimes cases occurred in which outside influences of a stronger kind manifested themselves. We quote two examples here. The first is taken from the *Fantasy in D flat major*, composed in 1913, the other from the piece entitled *Plaintive Sounds*, which was composed in the same

ness. It is for this reason that he follows his own line steadily, and does not allow himself, after the manner of many young composers, to come under the influence, by suggestion, of a variety of artistic schools whose aims do not coincide.

This is indeed a good sign, and was so especially at

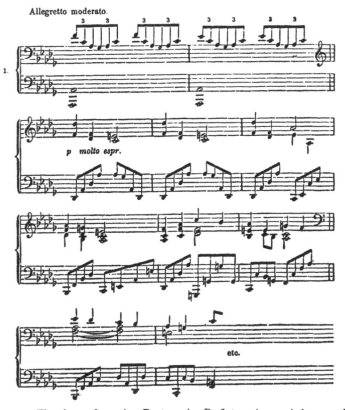

year. The theme from the *Fantasy in D flat major* reminds one of Chaminade. It appears to me that Erwin was in this case directly influenced by that author's *Pierrette*. The other theme was born under the influence of Chopin. In fact, the third and fourth bars appeared to me to be Chopin, pure and simple, but when I tried to trace them in the works of Chopin I

I

the time, when people were craving for originality, when there was a tendency to make a little talent go a long way by the use of far-fetched forms, and when the natural exaggerated affectation of a composer masqueraded as a valuable artistic asset. It stands to reason that in a period of art which aims at new ideas and new modes of expression, people will turn away from old models. Strong artistic personalities, who in such a period shape the course of artistic aspiration, will emancipate themselves from the traditions of the

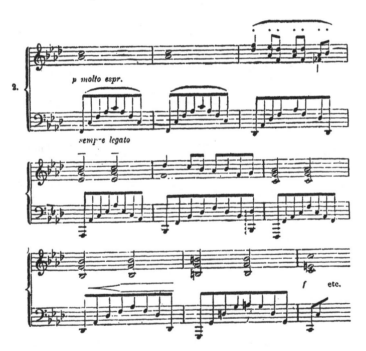

searched in vain. As regards feeling and character this theme, perhaps, most closely resembles the second theme (*sotto voce*) of the *B minor Nocturne* and of the *Prelude in F sharp major;* from a melodic point of view, it is closely related to the *Nocturne in D flat major* (comp. time 10-11).

past, as they speak a different language and are the bearers of new ideas and tendencies. They may not adopt the old forms, but they are none the less rooted in the past, whence they derived their artistic culture as well as their inspiration. So, in spite of their great independence they are also disciples, though in a different sense.

This, however, does not hold good for budding artists. In youth they are bound to lean upon somebody, till their ideas have assumed definite form. Artists belonging to a period closely connected with modern tendencies, though closed from the point of view of art, might serve this purpose better than the leaders of artistic movements still in a state of ferment.

For if the young artists possess great talents and are destined to open up new ways for art, they are bound to lay aside all that encumbers them in what they have learned. Anything of permanent value, however, in what they owe to their Great Masters, they will be careful to preserve and cherish. And though they may not always be successful in carrying out their ideas, they are in the vanguard of the new movement in art. Though they may sacrifice themselves for the sake of art in the preliminary struggle, to them belongs the credit of forming important intermediate links in the development of music.

The works of the Great Masters combine, in a

[1] These fundamental questions of movements in modern art are, among other works, treated by B. Alexander in a book valuable from a scientific as well as from a literary point of view, *L'Art*, Paris, 1914.

wonderful whole, all the modest and daring attempts of their predecessors; in fact, it may truly be said that they include everything that has ever been written or imagined.

My reason for considering that Erwin's musical taste is sound, and promises well for his future development, is based on the fact that a natural impulse prompts him to avoid those new schools in art, which are still imperfect and still in the course of development, and draw his inspiration from all that is most perfect in the past. As a follower of the classical school, he will do far better work, should his inclinations tend in the direction of modern art, than he would have achieved if he had followed this pioneer path in his youth.

In studying his compositions there is one characteristic which forces itself upon our notice. Each of his creations is individual, and has its own intrinsic mode of expression. Erwin's compositions are, at the same time, tender, powerful, placid, passionate, joyful, and melancholy. It is this that distinguishes him, in particular, from most "infant prodigies"; for these, in their first creative phase, are almost always monotonous in their portrayal of emotion. The small selection from Erwin's compositions which I publish here gives sufficient proof of the manner in which he differs in this respect. It is interesting to note that the characteristic richness and variety of his emotional writing struck Erwin himself, so much so that, on one occasion, he even alluded to it.

In addition to this diversity of expression, another

remarkable characteristic of his works is the unity of the emotional note which runs through each of his individual compositions. In fact, a fundamental note of emotion is sustained throughout each of his pieces. This shows, primarily, that each of them is the expression of an individual musical idea, and also that he never allows himself to be deterred from his purpose during execution, a point which deserves the highest commendation in so young a child.

As regards the fundamental note of expression in the individual compositions, it is usually lyrical, sometimes pathetic, and, in certain cases, dramatic, as in the *Moses Oratorio* and the *Fantasy*.

A means of expression of which he is very fond, and which perhaps serves to illustrate the romantic side of his character, is the contrast between depth and height. The whole range of the musical scale is employed in order to give colour to the melody. Examples of this may be found in the *Funeral March* for 'cello, the *Ballad*, and the *Cadenza*. The titles of the various pieces also are significant both of the certainty and directness with which he attacks the emotional side of music. In the selection of these he is infallible.

There are some who might argue that the emotions portrayed in the compositions are incompatible with the undeveloped character of a child, being confronted, on the one side, by a mere child with all his simple emotions, feelings, and desires, and, on the other, by his compositions, which are serious and full of meaning. They might find a discrepancy between his fine and emotional poetic soul and his childlike features.

But it is fundamentally wrong to assume that children do not possess a rich variety of feelings and emotions. It is easy not only to underrate the emotional life of children, and their own consciousness of it, but their capacity for introspection,[1] since, in their intercourse with grown-up people, they very often have little command of that most subtle of all means of expression —speech. They still use it clumsily, and they do not understand, as yet, either the complexities of expression, or the fine shades of accentuation. Besides, children do not, as a rule, give an account of their feelings and thoughts to others, for, owing to the shyness of youth, they have not the courage to do so. There are other reasons why their inner life is so veiled from us; for the most part their emotions are expressed in a different way from ours, and, above all, they lack the freedom, which we possess, of giving vent to our feelings by acts. It is very difficult to arrive at a thorough comprehension of the emotional life of a child, for this reason, if for no other, that a child behaves towards grown-up people like a snail, and if you touch it even on the surface it draws back into its shell. A child is usually distrustful of older people, and very rarely tells them about its hopes and expectations, therefore these remain hidden from them. But if, at any time, these feelings, emotions and desires see the light, we are

[1] I have had occasion to observe, in the case of a child five and a half years old, that it had learnt to observe, spontaneously, well-known, optical, subjective phenomena, as, for instance, positive and negative after-images, their phases, the conditions which favour their occurrence, the possibility of their projection, etc., and to describe them in a strikingly efficient way. (" Über spontane und systematische Selbstbeobachtung bei Kindern ", *Zeitschrift für angewandte Psychologie*, vol. 21, 1922.)

astonished at the depth and wealth of emotional experience which lie hidden in the child's soul, and we
realize how often we have misunderstood and under-
rated children, for the simple reason that we knew little
or nothing of the workings of their minds. But where
children have a gift for singing and music, it is a great
blessing, for they then possess a splendid medium for
the free and unhampered expression of their emotions,
and they reveal themselves in song and sound.

Another feature that distinguishes Erwin's compositions is their wealth of melody. This is a most
salient feature of his talent. In the first bloom of his
youth, when musical construction and form were still
undeveloped, he was driven to melody, and it took
possession of him altogether, streaming forth from the
deep well of his nature. And he actually achieved
originality in this respect, for all his melodies are
simple, natural, spontaneous, and fluid. They come
to us as they were conceived. And it is this simplicity,
spontaneity, and evident inspiration that marks the
genuineness and originality of his talent.

We cannot overestimate the terse manner in which
he works out his themes: he leads off with the chief
motif with no circumlocution, and he never draws out
anything longer than necessary at the end. This is
why most of his pieces appear so perfectly formed,
each of them is a finished picture, the proportions of
which are clear and easy to grasp.

There are occasions when another aspect of his
talent is particularly prominent, namely his feeling for
instrumental music. He has produced several com-

136 THE PSYCHOLOGY OF A MUSICAL PRODIGY

positions in which some parts suggest orchestral music, and are not particularly effective when played on the piano. This is all the more remarkable and significant of his future development as a composer, as, up to the time of the composition of these pieces, the only instrument he had played had been the piano. This peculiarity is very noticeable in an overture, composed in October 1911, an incomplete fragment in which, owing to the great number of independent parts, he was obliged to use three sets of lines. To this class the composition to which he has given the name of *Moses Oratorio* composed by him in his seventh year, and of which only a few fragments still exist, also belongs. The piece, which depicts the death of Moses, is a melancholy adagio, written in 4/4 time. The chief *motif* is brought out in a heavy and measured tempo, it is then varied a little, then transposed into the bass, where it loses itself, sinking into deep melancholy. Then a new phrase is introduced, treated quite as though he were writing for orchestra, slightly quicker in tempo, strongly marked, and full of vigour. The last chords (which he evidently felt as horns or trombones) lead to the final phrase in which the chief *motif* is heard in unison, in the lower register, pianissimo (contra-bass), increasing steadily in strength, then is carried once more to the dominant, in quicker tempo (orchestra with string instruments), until it melts away in the end.

In this composition he was inspired by the *Passion according to St Matthew*, which he had just heard. The whole piece sounds like the piano adaptation of an orchestral work. It is a matter for regret that it has not been written down, and was merely played by heart at the time by Erwin. I am, therefore, unable here to quote a work which is of interest also from other points of view.

Sometimes Erwin is so obsessed with the desire to express his musical ideas orchestrally that he over-steps the limit of technical possibilities on the piano. His remarkable ability for reading from the score, which I have already mentioned in a preceding chapter (p. 86), is also a proof of his strong feeling for orchestral music.

A talent for symphony-writing is clearly shown in a piece composed in 1914. The following fragment may serve as an example (see pp. 138, 139) :—

I should now like to add a few words on the subject of the progress of his development. This may be clearly seen in his works. The compositions printed here, although they represent only a very small portion of his productions up to now, give a very good idea of this development.

It may be assumed that, on the whole, Erwin made steady progress as a composer during his childhood, although the improvement was not always an even one. As in the case of his general mental develop-ment, lapses occurred which, at times, hampered the speed of his development. One of these manifested itself clearly between the seventh and eighth year of his age. The time at which this slowing down of his creative faculties (and probably also of his general musical capacity) occurred, coincides with the age at which the general mental development of a child is

From a *Dramatic Sonata*, 1914.

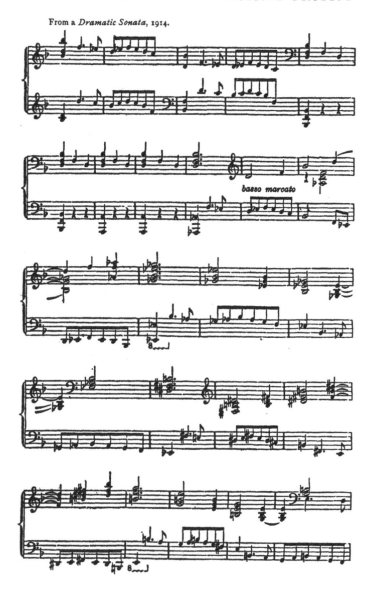

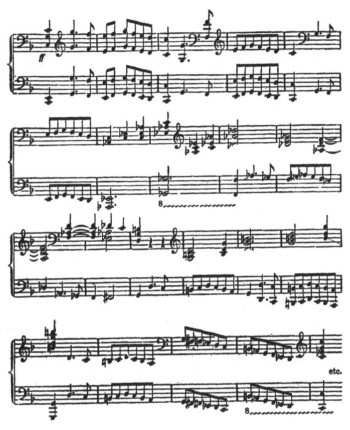

usually arrested, and it may be safely assumed that
both phenomena spring from a common cause. This
pause which we have observed in the development of
Erwin's talent as a composer may, therefore, be partly
ascribed to his physical growth, which increased
markedly at precisely this period. The well-known
reaction of physical growth upon the development of
the mind no doubt influenced the musical faculties
also. Probably school-work, to which at first he was

not accustomed, may also have had a detrimental effect upon his musical development.

Another possibility must also be taken into account when investigating this phenomenon. I have reason to believe that this rather prolonged delay may also be partly due to the fact that, during this period, Erwin had no musical help or inspiration, and did not even get a chance to enlarge his theoretical knowledge to any great extent. At that time, the only musical instruction he received was in piano playing, and it is not to be wondered at if owing to lack of fresh knowledge his musical development was arrested. As he learned nothing new, and received no personal guidance, he was obliged to content himself with such information as he had been able to acquire, helped by his extraordinary musicality and autodidactic receptivity, in his early childhood, and this was no longer sufficient for his increased wants; new matter and new forms were essential to him if his gift were to have a fair chance of developing further.

After his eighth, and even more noticeably after his ninth year, when his rapid bodily growth was more or less arrested, and his musical education was in full swing, his progress became very apparent, as may be clearly observed in the last three works published here.

In order to estimate the extent of his development, and, especially, with a view to studying the influence of musical instruction, I made him work out the same theme at different times. The theme was as follows :

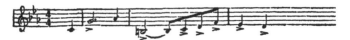

I gave him this theme and asked him to improvize on it. As soon as he had finished the improvization, I made him repeat it on the piano, and transcribe it. The first improvization dates from 1910 (June), the

Improvization dated 1910.

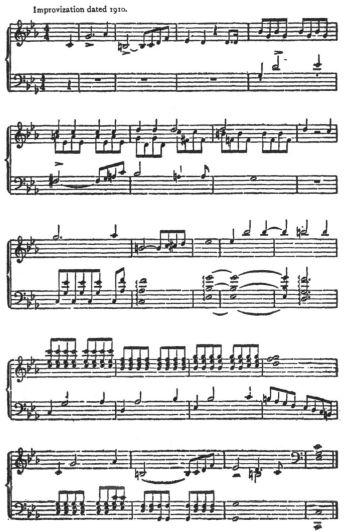

second from 1913 (also June). These two improvizations are important, not only as examples of Erwin's
musical development, but also as witnesses to his
spontaneity, his quickness of response, musically, and
the rapidity with which he worked.   The improvization
of 1913 took him under half an hour; this included the
time taken for writing it down and correcting it.

Improvization dated 1913.

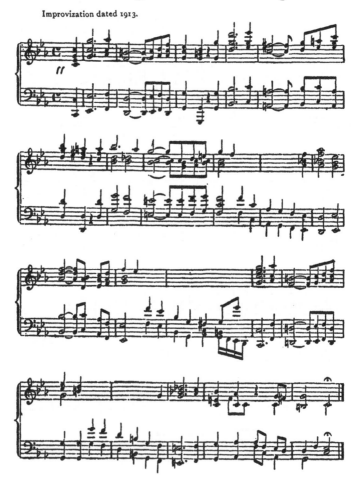

I publish a few of Erwin's compositions in the Appendix, in chronological order. I have altered nothing in the pieces but reproduce them exactly as they were composed by Erwin, and I have refrained from including works which have been corrected. I do not propose to give a precise analysis of the compositions, for every connoisseur will be able to recognize for himself the subtleties of expression, and construction, etc., without difficulty. I shall, therefore, content myself with sketching the character of the individual pieces in a few words, and drawing the reader's attention to the various important aspects of Erwin's talent as a composer as they manifested themselves as time went on.

The *Funeral March* for the 'cello, with piano accompaniment, is the earliest of the compositions published here. (Example No. 1.) It was composed during the summer of 1909, when Erwin was six and a half years old. At this time, he had not yet heard the 'cello played as a separate instrument, but only in the orchestra, a fact which makes the admirable manner in which he has adapted the whole piece to the character and range of the instrument all the more remarkable. With reference to this it is sufficient to designate the part, just before the close, in which the melody is taken into the higher octave, to emphasize its melancholy character. The piece is so well adapted to the instrument that, even in a transcription for the piano, it is obvious that it was originally written for the violoncello.

It would not be right to judge this composition from too technical a standpoint. We cannot expect conventional correctness of construction from a child of six, especially if he does not yet possess even an elementary knowledge of the theory of composition. The qualities which must be considered, in this instance, are power of invention and consistency in the portrayal of emotion. And, in this respect, Erwin achieved wonderful results for his age. If we disregard the laws of form, and the monotony of the piano accompaniment which, however, is quite in keeping with the character of a funeral march, and if we try, as we should in the case of a song, to fix our minds on the melody, always the most direct expression of sentiment, we cannot but feel that the soul of a poet has found expression in this rich, flowing air. Erwin's imagination is abundant and natural, he produces beautiful and inspired melodies, sometimes sustained, sometimes merely fragmentary. In spite of technical defects, a great portion of the composition shows a strong sense of form. The theme consisting of fifteen bars, at the beginning of the piece, is remarkable for this quality. Another part which is interesting is that marked "espressivo" and occurring just before the coda, for it corresponds perfectly to the rules of the simple form of a song. It consists, in fact, of two eight-bar periods, which is correct according to the rules.

One more observation—Erwin's compositions, as a rule, do not betray his Magyar descent. It might be possible to trace a Hungarian element in the *Funeral March*, for the first four bars have a familiar sound; the second two bars in particular are reminiscent of a popular song, but I have been unable to find any trace of the "Folk-Song" in any of his other compositions.

It would be greatly to the advantage of our national music if, later, Erwin were to base his art on the many beautiful and noble elements in Hungarian "Folk-Song."

The second work printed here, the *Serenata*, which is one of the loveliest of Erwin's creations, was composed in the year 1909, a few months after the *Funeral March*. (Example No. 2.) It is reminiscent of Mozart's day.

The *Serenata* appears to me to resemble the pianoforte compositions of Mozart when he was eight years old: it suggests them in its simplicity and depth of melody, consistency of musical expression and feeling, the treatment of the theme, and even as regards form. It is true that Mozart—as is apparent from his recently-published music-book[1] when eight years old—was a much more finished composer than Erwin, both from the point of view of form and, especially, of harmony— a fact that may be ascribed, not only to his far greater talent but, partly, to his exceptionally favourable musical surroundings, and the advanced musical education and culture of the period, which had so favourable an influence on the development of the musical talent of his day. In spite of this they have much in common, such as, for instance, the wealth of melody and unity of feeling, which both would seem to have possessed, if one compares the chronologically-corresponding compositions of the two children up to their seventh year of age.

[1] *Mozart als achtjähriger Komponist.* A music-book of Wolfgang, edited by Schünemann, Leipzig.

The melody of the *Serenata* is noble and harmonious : and is distinguished by its simplicity and spontaneity. The middle of the piece is remarkable, where it returns softly to the recurring chief *motif*, and the beautiful treatment of the figure appearing in the third bar, is specially noticeable.

From a technical point of view, the *Serenata* is much more finished than the *Funeral March*. It represents a simple song in sections of three parts.

About the same time as the *Serenata* Erwin composed a *Ballad*. In this composition he wished to try his hand at bigger things. In spite of its deficiencies, this *Ballad* must be looked upon as a work of particular interest. It consists of a string of melodies in close relation to each other, which, by the consistency of their underlying emotional idea are merged into a continuous musical impression. In this *Ballad* one is struck by the fact that, in contrast to former works, a certain interest in technical execution is shown. This is specially indicated by certain passages which, at first hearing, sound a little trivial, but which improve on acquaintance. The piece would certainly arouse interest if it could be published in full, but it is too long (two hundred and four bars). Therefore, to my regret, I was obliged to omit it altogether.

The next example is a *Night Song*, also composed in 1909 (Example No. 3). Its chief characteristic is its change of rhythm. From the fifteenth to the nineteenth bars it is reminiscent of a Hungarian popular song. I only give the first part of the piece here, as the rest merely contains insignificant modifications of the theme.

Further progress is apparent in the *Tema con varia-zioni*, composed in 1910 (Example No. 4). The theme chosen is simple, consisting of eight bars, and is very well adapted to variation. Although the composition has no great claim to originality, as an artistic feat it merits attention. We find a new quality of Erwin's in the variations, namely a strong sense of rhythm. This sense of rhythm and the absolute certainty both in tempo and metre, is particularly apparent in his piano playing. It is interesting to note the manner in which a change of rhythm is used as a means of variation. As the variations themselves are not particularly indicative of the progress of the child, I only give the theme, and a few short variations.

It was in the same year that Erwin composed his *Spring Song* (Example No. 5). It is a tender, pure, and fragrant melody. The principal theme is most successful, whereas the middle section (not given here) lacks vigour. Although it is perhaps not quite original (it is reminiscent of Mendelssohn), it shows marked power of invention. It also manifests signs of technical progress. Erwin, who had not then had any instruction in the theory of composition, has written it in the conventional form of a three-part song.

From his output in the following year, 1911, I should like to quote one work (Example No. 6). This is a *Cadenza*, which he composed to Haydn's *Concerto in D major* (*opus* 21). The occasion arose when he was asked to perform this piece at a pupils' concert. He had already observed, on looking through the pages of the *Concerto* for the first time, that the *Cadenza* in

Steingräber's edition could not possibly be the work of Haydn, and when he afterwards learnt that it was customary to compose one's own Cadenza to this piece, he determined to write one himself.

The *Cadenza* is based on the first two bars of the following principal theme of the *Concerto* :

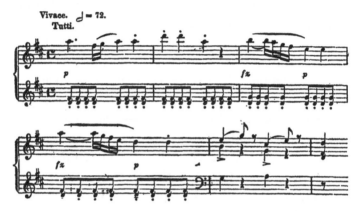

As may be seen in the Appendix, the *Cadenza* is a development of this *motif* of two bars. The theme is amplified brilliantly and effectively, and is developed in a masterly manner. Its treatment is witness to the enormous strides Erwin had made in his musical education, and is the result of the lessons in harmony he had received during the past few months.[1] The way in which the *Cadenza* is worked out serves to prove how easily one may be led astray, in judging the compositions of children, by attributing too great importance to lack of form and faulty construction. We see here, with what little trouble Erwin mastered the

[1] At that time, Erwin had already studied the greater part of the theory of harmony.

difficulties that had beset him in his earlier work, how correctly he had already begun, in many cases, to modulate, and how by degrees he arrived at an understanding of counterpoint.

Another point to be taken into account in connection with this work is the zeal with which it was composed, the entire piece being written in the course of two days. Erwin does not count the *Cadenza* among his most successful achievements; in fact, he never mentions it at all. He looks upon it merely as a kind of exercise, having been hampered in the full flow of his imagination by the alien theme and the fact that he was being made to write with an object.

I regret to say that the *Cadenza* had already been revised and corrected as regards harmony, when I saw it. The corrections, however—so his teacher assures me—were insignificant.

In the year 1912 the boy's time was so much taken up with his education that he found little time for composing. In spite of this fact he wrote, as well as a quantity of exercises, a considerable number of original pieces. Of these, I have selected a *Scherzo* (Example No. 7). As the principal theme we find a pretty, fresh, scherzo *motif*. The second part of the piece develops the same theme, according to the rules of counterpoint. Then follows a short piece in the middle (a transition), which is modulated back into the principal theme. I only give the principal *motif* here for the special purpose of showing how admirably adapted it is to the character of a scherzo.

From the output of 1913 I give three compositions:

two small and one large one. All three were composed in the spring.

I wish to emphasize these pieces in particular, because they illustrate the general progress Erwin had made. They are clearer and more perfect in form, richer and more correct as regards harmonies, and the part-writing is better worked out. Erwin had matured and become more thoughtful, a fact that is shown by his avoidance of insignificant things, *naïvetés* and banalities, such as, for instance, meaningless phrases and transitions. It was as though he realized that genuine artistic creation was too noble a thing to permit of the use of soulless decorations.

Of the works produced in 1913 I consider that the *Theme* (also called *Longing*) is the finest (Example No. 8). In spite of a slight reminiscence of Schumann, I find it original. In this piece we are struck by Erwin's musical knowledge, his fine taste, and strong sense of form, and, behind these, lies such power that the theme would do credit even to an adult composer, though, it must be admitted, only to one belonging to an earlier period. In this composition Erwin has reached perfection in a small compass. He has expressed what he wished to say concisely, and without unnecessary circumlocution, and one would not wish either to add or omit anything.

The reader should note the expressive melody, which advances, quietly but boldly, from the depths to the heights; the middle of the piece which, with its energetic, resounding notes, gives an impression of strength and austerity; the exaltation of the bar before the last in this portion ; and, finally, the close, which dies away into silence.

Simplicity, freshness, spontaneity, and purity of technique characterize the *Second Spring Song*, composed at the same time (Example No. 9). Erwin's power of invention is not so striking here as in the *Serenata*, and the artistic quality of the development is less obvious than in the *Theme ;* but the playful ease and the uniformity with which the song is wafted forth mark the fine musician, and the inspiration is that of a poet. The melody is fresh and joyful ; it is redolent of the air of spring ; and one becomes familiar with it so quickly that it almost seems like the echo of some well-known air.

Besides these two pieces Erwin wrote a *Fantasy* (Example No. 10) in the spring of 1913. This, it is true, owing to its great length, is less uniform in character than the two last-named pieces, but it is remarkable for its masterly development, and for its "orchestral" quality.

Nature had certainly endowed Erwin with wonderful gifts, but, at the time, his powers were not sufficiently developed, or his musical education far enough advanced for it to be possible for him to create anything great on a large scale. Any big work he might produce would, therefore, necessarily be of a rhapsodical character and would seem to be lacking in unity as a whole.

As regards its form, the *Fantasy* consists of seven parts and a coda. The chief *motif* appears in the first two bars of the first section ; is treated in a quiet, serious, pathetic manner, and establishes the fundamental note of the whole piece. It is not impossible that this *motif* was borrowed from the finale of the *C minor Sonata* by Beethoven (*opus* 10, No. 1); but, in Erwin's work, the first four bars of Beethoven's theme were carried out in an altered rhythm, in another kind of metre, and in a different tempo. The development of the *motif*, however, and its general character are so fundamentally different from that of Beethoven that it is more than probable that Erwin evolved the theme quite independently. The second section, which is closely related to, and seems to be a mere development of the first, advances with great strength and vitality, and is reinforced by the lofty, but rather monotonous treatment of the bass. The climax comes with an arpeggio. Then a short new *motif* appears, which, however, soon proves to be the transition to a new theme. This theme helps the chief *motif* to new life, but does not give it sufficient depth. The chief theme, indeed, appears several times, in various forms, in this and the following part, but is not treated thematically. The whole of the middle part, from the thirty-second bar to the seventy-ninth, makes the composition of the whole piece difficult to grasp, and disturbs its equilibrium. But, for us, this middle part is interesting, because it shows the dexterity and ease with which Erwin was able to amplify and use the technical knowledge he had acquired during the past year owing, chiefly, to his study of harmony. The repetition of the principal subject in the last movement is, perhaps, its most interesting feature from a musical point of view.

It breathes storm and passion ; nowhere else has Erwin made use of sound to this extent.   His aim was the repetition of the principal subject in an expressive manner ; therefore he forced the climax until the end, wishing to attain the utmost heights of exaltation.   To get this effect, he used a strong bass, increasing in volume and carrying the whole movement, fortissimo, to the climax. I must, however, confess that, in spite of its good qualities which, in my opinion, are technical rather than creative, I find, in this work, less originality, clearness, and spontaneity than in Erwin's earlier and more successful pieces.

Among the compositions he produced in and about his eleventh year, there are three remarkable pieces ; a *Fantasy in D flat major*, one in F sharp minor, and a piece called *Plaintive Sounds*.

Of these compositions the last is the most interesting and best deserves our attention.   It consists of three parts, which, indeed, have no real connection with each other, but which are united by the spirit of melancholy that inspires them all.   I give the first theme only here, in which the child's style of invention and harmonization, in short, his present artistic level, is shown at its best (Example No. 11).   It is well known that the *motif* B flat—A—C—B has already been made the subject of a famous fugue by Bach in his *Art of Fugue;* and that, later on, it was employed both by Schumann and by Liszt. Whether Erwin's compositions owe anything to the influence of these compositions is an open question. As to the third theme, which is reminiscent of Chopin, I have already published it on p. 130.

These two fantasies are developed in a virtuoso style. As in Erwin's earlier compositions, we are struck by the gift for melody, the rich inventive power, the taste, and the manly, open character of the child. All his themes are striking, simple, short, and only rarely verbose. And though, already, certain outside influences may be increasingly discernible in them, as, for instance, in the principal theme of the *Fantasy in D flat major*, they may still be considered the independent creations of a rare poetic spirit. As, however, they do not strike me as particularly characteristic of either the musical talent or the development of Erwin, I have not quoted them.

The last manuscript he sent me was a piece for the piano in Sonata form, which he composed in the spring of 1914. As I find this piece significant of his progress as a composer, and as it also appears to me to show the standard of his work at that time, I include its best part, the " Adagio " here (Example No. 12). This, I consider, completes my record of his creative activity up to the end of his eleventh year.

Of his further development as a composer I regret to say I know nothing. Erwin has left Europe, and in consequence I have lost touch with him. How he has progressed during this critical period of his musical development, I cannot say ; I can only hope, however, that his great talent will enable him to pass through it unscathed, and that ephemeral and sensational success will not afford him lasting satisfaction.

12. Progress of Erwin's Creative Musical Development as shown in his Works.

Example 1.

FUNERAL MARCH.　(For Violoncello and Piano.)

Composed at the age of 7.　(Summer, 1909.)

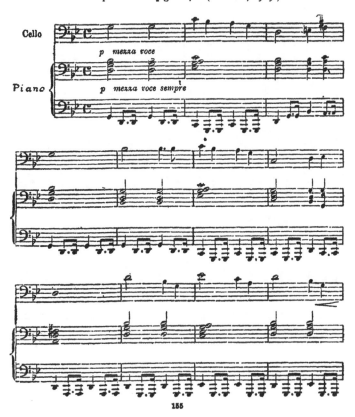

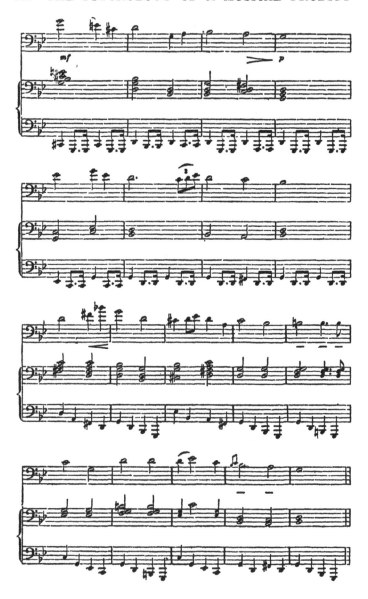

Example 2.

SERENATA.

Composed at the age of 7. (September 1909.)

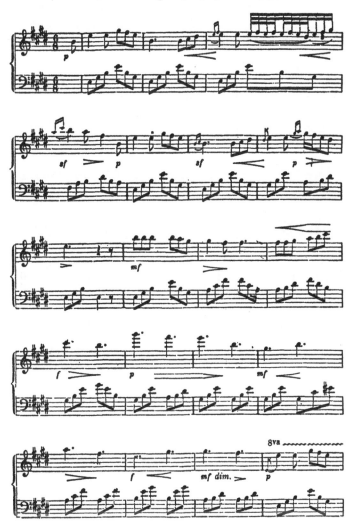

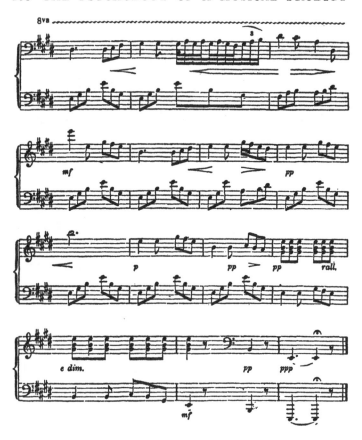

Example 3.

NIGHT SONG.

Composed at the age of 7. (October 1909.)

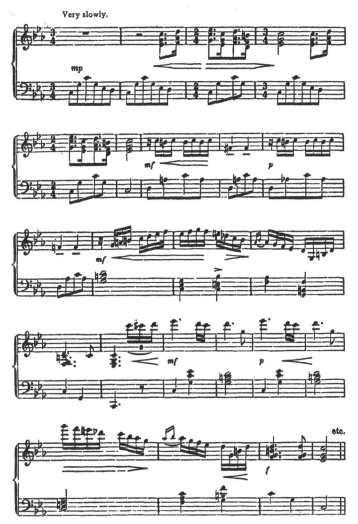

Example 4.

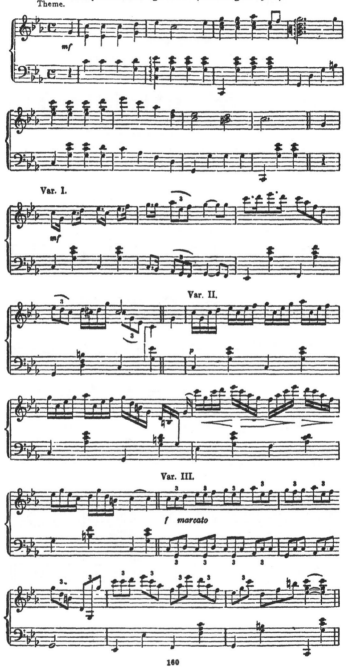

VARIATIONS ON AN ORIGINAL THEME.
Composed at the age of 8.   (11th August 1910.)

Example 5.

SPRING SONG.

Composed at the age of 8.   (November 1910.)

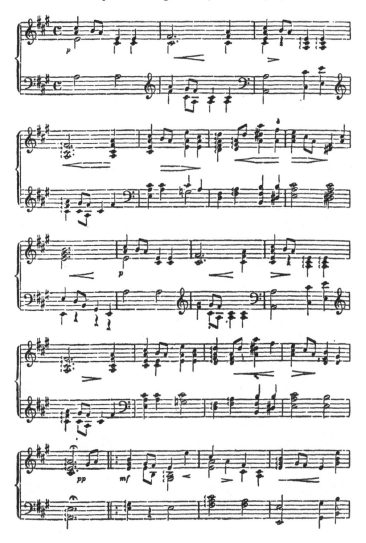

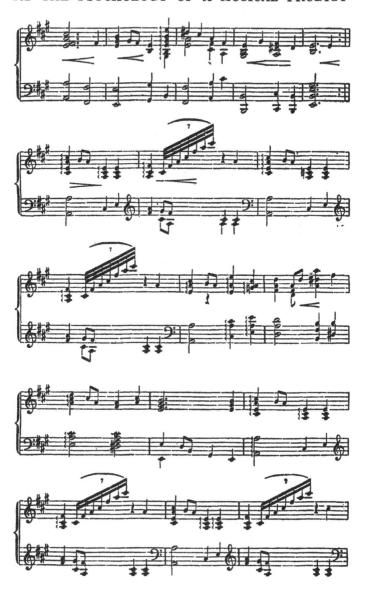

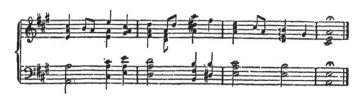

Example 6.

CADENZA FOR THE PIANO-CONCERTO D MAJOR.
J. HAYDN. (OP. 21.)

Composed at the age of 9. (October 1911.)

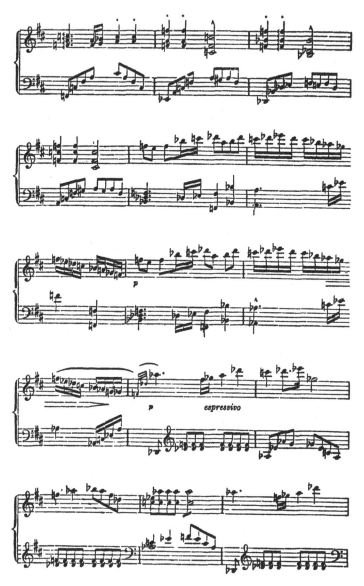

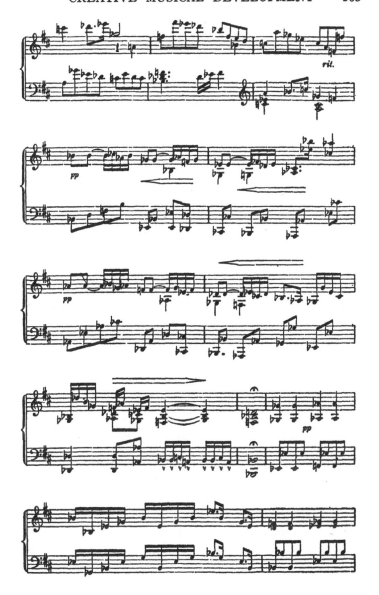

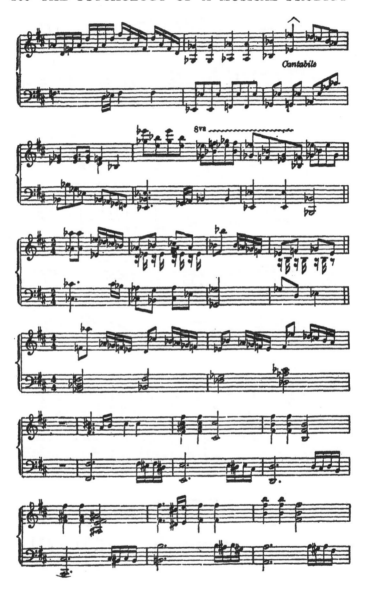

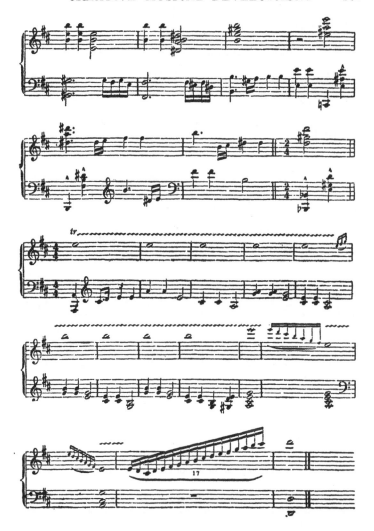

Example 7.

SCHERZO.

Composed at the age of 9.   (November 1912)

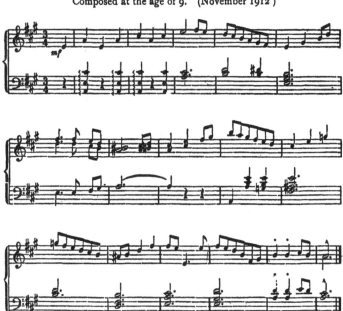

Example 8.

THEME (LONGING).

Composed at the age of 11.   (April 1913.)

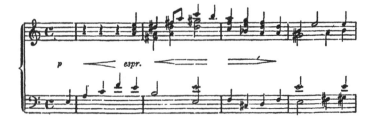

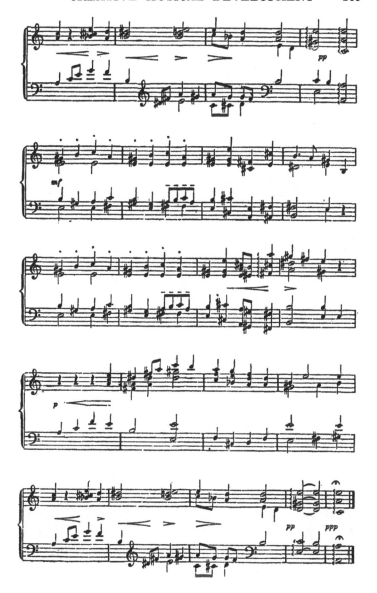

Example 9.

SPRING SONG.

Composed at the age of 11. (April 1913.)

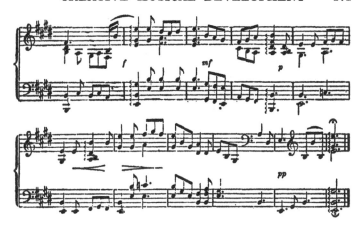

Example 10.

FANTASY.

Composed at the age of 11.   (May 1913.)

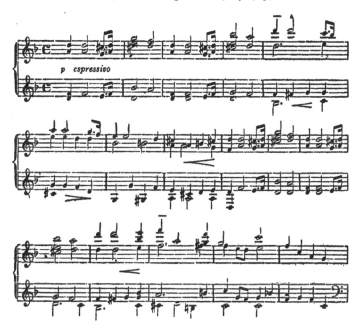

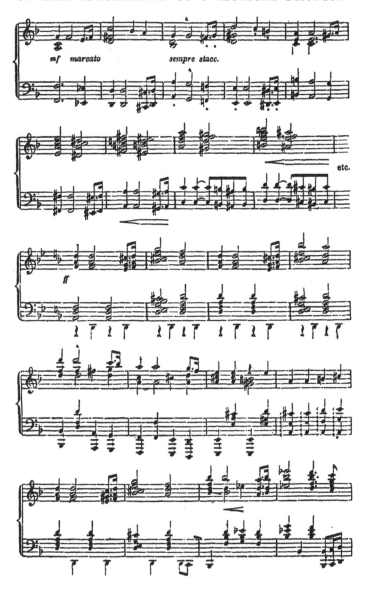

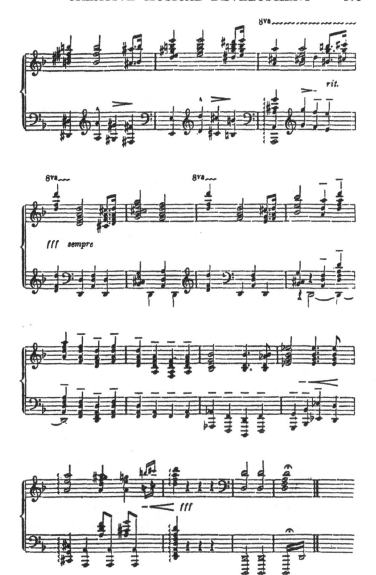

Example 11.

PLAINTIVE SOUNDS.

Composed at the age of 11. (September 1913.)

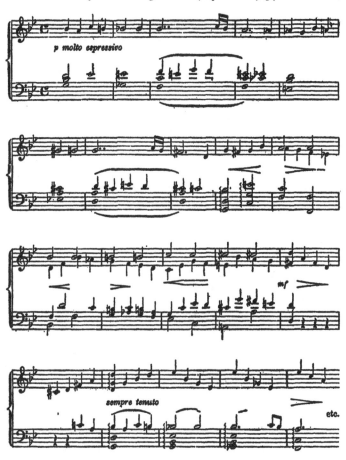

Example 12.

ADAGIO FROM A DRAMATIC SONATA.
Composed at the age of 12.   (April 1914.)

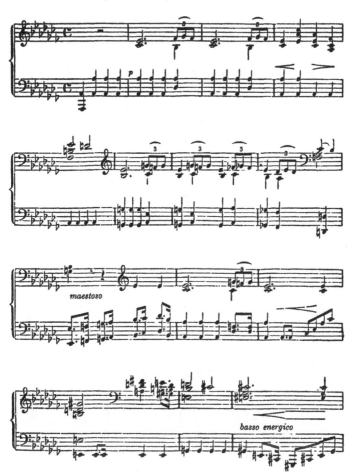

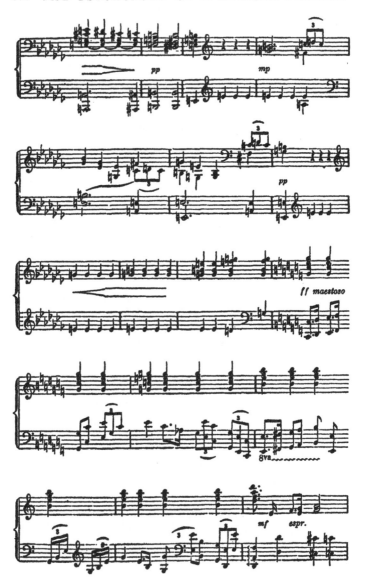

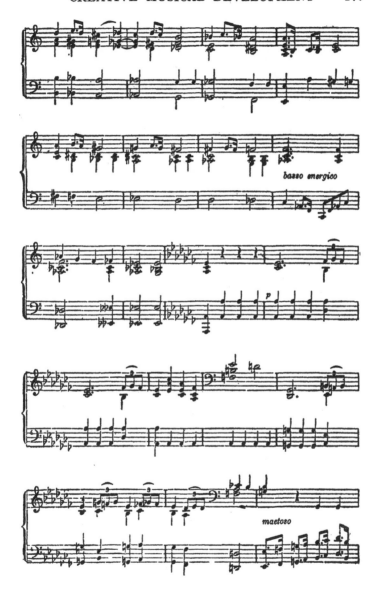

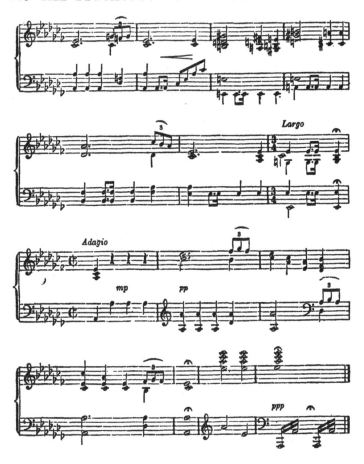

INDEX